Primary Immunodeficiency Disorders

Editor

LISA J. KOBRYNSKI

IMMUNOLOGY AND ALLERGY CLINICS OF NORTH AMERICA

www.immunology.theclinics.com

Consulting Editor
STEPHEN A. TILLES

February 2019 • Volume 39 • Number 1

ELSEVIER

1600 John F. Kennedy Boulevard • Suite 1800 • Philadelphia, Pennsylvania, 19103-2899
http://www.theclinics.com

IMMUNOLOGY AND ALLERGY CLINICS OF NORTH AMERICA Volume 39, Number 1
February 2019 ISSN 0889-8561, ISBN-13: 978-0-323-65441-8

Editor: Jessica McCool
Developmental Editor: Kristen Helm

Immunology and Allergy Clinics of North America (ISSN 0889–8561) is published quarterly by Elsevier Inc., 360 Park Avenue South, New York, NY 10010-1710. Months of issue are February, May, August, and November. Periodicals postage paid at New York, NY and additional mailing offices. Subscription prices are $341.00 per year for US individuals, $593.00 per year for US institutions, $100.00 per year for US students and residents, $423.00 per year for Canadian individuals, $220.00 per year for Canadian students, $753.00 per year for Canadian institutions, $447.00 per year for international individuals, $753.00 per year for international institutions, $220.00 per year for international students. To receive student/resident rate, orders must be accompanied by name of affiliated institution, date of term, and the *signature* of program/residency coordinator on institution letterhead. Orders will be billed at individual rate until proof of status is received. Foreign air speed delivery is included in all *Clinics* subscription prices. All prices are subject to change without notice. **POSTMASTER:** Send address changes to *Immunology and Allergy Clinics of North America,* Elsevier Health Sciences Division, Subscription Customer Service, 3251 Riverport Lane, Maryland Heights, MO 63043. **Customer Service: 1-800-654-2452 (U.S. and Canada); 314-447-8871 (outside U.S. and Canada). Fax: 314-447-8029. E-mail: journalscustomerservice-usa@elsevier.com (for print support); journalsonlinesupport-usa@elsevier.com (for online support).**

Reprints. For copies of 100 or more, of articles in this publication, please contact the Commercial Reprints Department, Elsevier Inc., 360 Park Avenue South, New York, New York 10010-1710. Tel. 212-633-3874, Fax: 212-633-3820, E-mail: reprints@elsevier.com.

Immunology and Allergy Clinics of North America is covered in MEDLINE/PubMed (Index Medicus), Current Contents/Life Sciences, Science Citation Index, ISI/BIOMED, Chemical Abstracts, and EMBASE/Excerpta Medica.

Contributors

CONSULTING EDITOR

STEPHEN A. TILLES, MD
Executive Director, ASTHMA Inc Clinical Research Center, Partner, Northwest Asthma and Allergy Center, Clinical Professor of Medicine, University of Washington, Seattle, Washington, USA

EDITOR

LISA J. KOBRYNSKI, MD, MPH
Associate Professor of Pediatrics, Marcus Professor of Immunology, Section of Allergy/Immunology, Emory University, Atlanta, Georgia, USA

AUTHORS

SHRADHA AGARWAL, MD
Associate Professor of Medicine, Icahn School of Medicine at Mount Sinai, New York, New York, USA

VINCENT R. BONAGURA, MD
Jack Hausman Professor of Pediatrics, Professor of Molecular Medicine, Donald and Barbara Zucker School of Medicine at Hofstra/Northwell, Chief, Division of Allergy/Immunology, Northwell Health System, Division of Allergy, Asthma and Immunology, Great Neck, New York, USA

LORI BRODERICK, MD, PhD
Division of Allergy, Immunology and Rheumatology, Assistant Professor, Department of Pediatrics, University of California, San Diego, La Jolla, California, USA

SHANMUGANATHAN CHANDRAKASAN, MD
Division of Bone Marrow Transplant, Aflac Cancer and Blood Disorders Center, Children's Healthcare of Atlanta, Emory University School of Medicine, Atlanta, Georgia, USA

CHARLOTTE CUNNINGHAM-RUNDLES, MD, PhD
Professor of Medicine and Pediatrics, The David S. Gottesman Professor, The Icahn School of Medicine at Mount Sinai, The Immunology Institute, New York, New York, USA

MORNA J. DORSEY, MD, MMSc
Department of Pediatrics, University of California, San Francisco, San Francisco, California, USA

JENNA R.E. BERGERSON, MD, MPH
Laboratory of Clinical Immunology and Microbiology, National Institutes of Allergy and Infectious Diseases (NIAID), National Institutes of Health (NIH), Bethesda, Maryland, USA

ALEXANDRA F. FREEMAN, MD
Laboratory of Clinical Immunology and Microbiology, National Institutes of Allergy and Infectious Diseases (NIAID), National Institutes of Health (NIH), Bethesda, Maryland, USA

JENNIFER HEIMALL, MD
Assistant Professor of Clinical Pediatrics, Division of Allergy and Immunology, Perelman School of Medicine at University of Pennsylvania, The Children's Hospital of Philadelphia, Philadelphia, Pennsylvania

BLANKA KAPLAN, MD
Assistant Professor of Medicine and Pediatrics at Donald and Barbara Zucker School of Medicine at Hofstra/Northwell, Director, Drug Allergy and Desensitization Center, Northwell Health System, Division of Allergy, Asthma and Immunology, Great Neck, New York, USA

JUDITH R. KELSEN, MD
Division of Gastroenterology, Hepatology and Nutrition, Philadelphia, Pennsylvania, USA

JENNIFER M. PUCK, MD
Department of Pediatrics, University of California, San Francisco, San Francisco, California, USA

PIERRE RUSSO, MD
Department of Pathology, The Children's Hospital of Philadelphia, Philadelphia, Pennsylvania, USA

ODED SHAMRIZ, MD
Division of Bone Marrow Transplant, Aflac Cancer and Blood Disorders Center, Children's Healthcare of Atlanta, Emory University School of Medicine, Atlanta, Georgia, USA; Pediatric Division, Hadassah-Hebrew University Medical Center, Jerusalem, Israel

KATHLEEN E. SULLIVAN, MD, PhD
Division of Allergy Immunology, The Children's Hospital of Philadelphia, Philadelphia, Pennsylvania, USA

RICHARD L. WASSERMAN, MD, PhD
Medical Director of Pediatric Allergy and Immunology, Medical City Children's Hospital, Managing Partner, Allergy Partners of North Texas, Dallas, Texas

Contents

In the United States, significant improvement in diagnosis and outcomes for children affected with severe combined immunodeficiency has followed institution of newborn screening using an assay to measure T-cell receptor excision circles in newborn dried blood spot specimens. Key to this outcome is the avoidance of infectious complications in infants with severe combined immunodeficiency.

The autoinflammatory diseases encompass approximately 30 monogenic disorders in which inborn errors in the innate immune system lead to episodic systemic inflammation. Largely mediated by dysregulation of myeloid cells, interleukin (IL)-1β, type I interferon, and NF-κB, these disorders have rapidly expanded over the past several years, and increasing numbers of patients identified. Crossover disorders, bridging autoinflammation and immunodeficiency, have recently been described. This article focuses on the clinical presentation of IL-1 and interferon-driven autoinflammatory disorders, and discusses novel diseases with features of immunodeficiency. Approaches to the clinical diagnosis, genetic testing, and treatment of these disorders are addressed.

Secondary hypogammaglobulinemia is an increasingly common development in patients treated with immunomodulatory agents for autoimmune, connective tissue and malignant diseases. It has also been observed in the medical management of patients undergoing stem cell and solid organ transplantation. Some patients have preexisting immunodeficiency, associated with these illnesses and immunosuppressive treatment magnifies their immune defect. This manuscript reviews immunosuppressive medications, including biologic treatments that cause secondary hypogammaglobulinemia. It summarizes risk factors for rituximab-induced

Hematopoietic stem cell transplantation (HSCT) in patients with primary immunodeficiency disorders (PIDDs) is being increasingly used as a curative option. Understanding the critical components, such as disease's nature and activity and pre-HSCT and post-HSCT patient care is key to a successful outcome. HSCT should be tailored to the underlying PIDD, as different PIDDs, such as severe combined immune deficiency, Treg dysfunction, and phagocytic disorders, have different transplant approaches. Therefore, successful HSCT in patients with PIDDs requires teamwork between immunologists and transplant physicians. In this article, the authors elaborate on various aspects of PIDD-HSCT and highlight recent advances.

Since the first genes associated with primary immunodeficiency were described in the early 1990s, there has been an exponential increase in the number of genes found to have pathologic variants in patients with symptoms of primary immunodeficiency. Genetic testing currently used clinically includes chromosomal microarray, Sanger sequencing, and next-generation sequencing techniques, including whole exome testing. With the knowledge of the underlying molecular pathways, biologic therapies have been used for treatment and efforts are underway to broaden the availability of gene therapy.

IMMUNOLOGY AND ALLERGY CLINICS OF NORTH AMERICA

THE CLINICS ARE AVAILABLE ONLINE!
Access your subscription at:
www.theclinics.com

Foreword

Diagnosis and Management of Primary Immunodeficiency Disorders: The Pieces of the Puzzle Are Starting to Fit Together

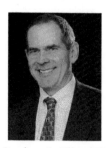

Stephen A. Tilles, MD
Consulting Editor

Not too many years ago many, practicing allergists viewed primary immunodeficiency disorders (PIDD) as a group of rare diseases with unknown underlying genetic defects, which were diagnosed based primarily on clinical presentation combined with rudimentary laboratory testing. With few exceptions, available treatments were unsatisfactory as well. In fact, despite realizing that real patients were suffering from these diseases, for many of us the world of PIDD was primarily of interest as a way of helping us understand how the immune system works.

Well, times have changed. Thanks to the efforts by scores of dedicated basic and clinical scientists, the world of PIDD has evolved into one of enhanced understanding and promising treatments. More importantly, lives are being saved, and this is especially noteworthy given that diseases affecting small numbers of patients are often neglected. For example, recounting and comparing stories of the most severe combined immune deficiency (SCID) patients just two decades ago compared with today is nothing short of remarkable.

In this issue of the *Immunology and Allergy Clinics of North America*, Editor Lisa J. Kobrynski has organized a series of reviews that update us on the PIDD world, including newborn screening for SCID, advances in genetic testing leading to improvements in the lives of patients, recently recognized syndromes that involve elevations in IgE, and advances in hematopoietic transplantation. There is also a fascinating article emphasizing new personalized approaches to administering immunoglobulin replacement therapy.

Immunol Allergy Clin N Am 39 (2019) ix–x
https://doi.org/10.1016/j.iac.2018.09.002
0889-8561/19/© 2018 Published by Elsevier Inc.

immunology.theclinics.com

I highly recommend this issue of the *Immunology and Allergy Clinics of North America* as an informative reference for all practicing Allergy/Immunology specialists and other physicians and caregivers who help take care of patients with PIDD.

Stephen A. Tilles, MD
ASTHMA Inc Clinical Research Center
Northwest Asthma and Allergy Center
University of Washington
9725 3rd Avenue Northeast, Suite 500
Seattle, WA 98115, USA

E-mail address:
stilles@nwasthma.com

Preface

Primary Immunodeficiency Disorders

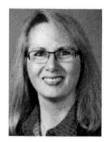

Lisa J. Kobrynski, MD, MPH
Editor

This issue on primary immunodeficiency disorders (PIDD) builds upon a previous set of reviews in the *Immunology and Allergy Clinics of North America*. The field of Clinical Immunology continues to expand at a rapid rate, so this issue updates readers on new diagnoses and new therapies and highlights some of the exciting developments in our field. Many of our well-known colleagues have contributed their expertise and time to educate us about important advances, which will benefit our patients with PIDD.

Beginning with diagnosis, the article on newborn screening for Severe Combined Immunodeficiency (SCID) demonstrates the success of this program, available in nearly the entire country, using population screening performed at birth, to detect this usually fatal PIDD. Previously, only a few infants were diagnosed prior to the onset of symptoms. Drs Puck and Dorsey discuss the rationale and benefits of newborn screening for SCID, highlighting the impact of early testing on patient outcomes. Then, we discuss two immune deficiencies, hereditary autoinflammatory disorders and secondary hypogammaglobulinemia, which are becoming increasingly common, but can often present challenges in diagnosis and treatment. Dr Lori Broderick discusses diagnosis and treatment of monogeneic disorders causing fever, inflammation, and other symptoms, while Drs Bonagura and Kaplan review the risk factors for secondary hypogammaglobulinemia, which can be a complication of both underlying disease and its treatment.

New phenotypes have been described for several disorders, and we feel that recognition of these presentations will aid in diagnosis. Dr Freeman discusses recently recognized syndromes, besides STAT loss-of-function (hyperIgE syndrome), associated with elevations in serum IgE. Early onset inflammatory bowel disease is now known to have several monogeneic causes and is a new addition to the family of PIDDs. Dr Sullivan informs readers of the recognition of these alternate presentations

Immunol Allergy Clin N Am 39 (2019) xi–xii
https://doi.org/10.1016/j.iac.2018.09.001
0889-8561/19/© 2018 Published by Elsevier Inc.

of PIDD. This can lead to early diagnosis and initiation of treatment. In addition, many PIDD frequently have difficult-to-treat complications that lead to significant morbidity and mortality. Drs Cunningham-Rundles and Agarwal review "Gastrointestinal Manifestations and Complications of Primary Immunodeficiency Disorders," focusing on clinical and pathologic clues to diagnosis as well as some potential therapies.

We are fortunate that therapies for PIDD and their complications continue to evolve and improve. Personalized medicine utilizes our understanding of the mechanisms of disease to inform predictions of response to specific therapies, allowing us to tailor our therapeutic approach to each individual patient. We see examples of this in the reviews on "Personalized Therapy: Immunoglobulin Replacement for Antibody Deficiency," by Dr Wasserman, and an "Update on Advances in Hematopoietic Cell Transplantation for Primary Immunodeficiency Disorders," by Drs Chandrakasan and Shamriz.

Last, we go back to the beginning, by reviewing genome testing for diagnosis of PIDD. Dr Heimall describes the benefits and limitations of genetic testing as well as the implications for treatment of PIDD. Since many therapeutic decisions are now dependent upon making a precise diagnosis and identifying the underlying molecular defect, it is more important than ever that we feel confident in the use of genetic testing.

We hope that the articles in this issue review and add to our knowledge, leading to improvements in the diagnosis and care of patients with PIDD. Our aim is to provide practitioners with clinically relevant information that can advance the care of these often complex patients.

Lisa J. Kobrynski, MD, MPH
Section, Allergy/Immunology
Emory University
2015 Uppergate Dr
Atlanta, GA 30322, USA

E-mail address:
lkobryn@emory.edu

Newborn Screening for Severe Combined Immunodeficiency in the United States: Lessons Learned

Morna J. Dorsey, MD, MMSc[a],*, Jennifer M. Puck, MD[b]

KEYWORDS

- Severe combined immunodeficiency (SCID) • Newborn screen (NBS)
- T-cell receptor excision circles (TRECs) • Hematopoietic cell transplant (HCT)
- T-cell lymphopenia

KEY POINTS

- Newborn screening for severe combined immunodeficiency is effective for identifying severe combined immunodeficiency.
- Early diagnosis of severe combined immunodeficiency leads to improved outcomes.
- In addition to diagnosing severe combined immunodeficiency, screening of newborns for low T-cell receptor excision circles has identified non–severe combined immunodeficiency T-cell lymphopenia.

INTRODUCTION

Improved outcomes in severe combined immunodeficiency (SCID) affected children are associated with early identification. The assay measuring T-cell receptor

Funding Sources: M.J. Dorsey received support from R01 GM107132 and The Michelle Platt-Ross Foundation; J.M. Puck received support from R01 AI105776; U54 AI082973 for the Primary Immune Deficiency Treatment Consortium, a member of the Rare Diseases Clinical Research Network (RDCRN) funded by the NIAID and ORDR, NCATS, NIH; The Jeffrey Modell Foundation and The Michelle Platt-Ross Foundation.
Financial Disclosures: The authors have indicated they have no financial relationships relevant to this article to disclose.
Potential Conflicts of Interest: J.M. Puck discloses spousal employment at a clinical DNA sequencing company, Invitae.
[a] Department of Pediatrics, University of California San Francisco, 555 Mission Bay Boulevard South, San Francisco, CA 94158, USA; [b] Department of Pediatrics, University of California San Francisco, Box 3118, 555 Mission Bay Boulevard South, Rm SC-252K, San Francisco, CA 94143, USA
* Corresponding author. Department of Pediatrics, Division of Allergy, Immunology and Bone Marrow Transplantation, University of California San Francisco, Box 0434, 550 16th Street, 4th Floor, San Francisco, CA 94143-0107.
E-mail address: Morna.Dorsey@ucsf.edu

excision circles (TRECs) in newborn dried blood spot specimens has revolutionized the ability to detect SCID in its presymptomatic phase and, therefore, led to improved outcomes. Implementation of population-wide SCID newborn screening (NBS) was piloted in 2008 in Wisconsin. Following the recommendation in 2010 to add this to the Recommended Uniform Screening Panel, SCID NBS has been widely adopted, with 48 states and Puerto Rico routinely screening all newborns as of July 2018 (**Fig. 1**).[1] TREC NBS for SCID permits identification of infants with SCID and a number of other T-cell lymphopenia (TCL) disorders before the development of infections and other complications. It has also paved the way for future use of DNA-based population screening, including the use of gene panels or whole exome and genome sequencing.

BIOLOGY OF SEVERE COMBINED IMMUNODEFICIENCY

SCID is a group of disorders characterized by profound impairment in T-cell development and function and also having no specific antibody production.[2–5] Normal T-cell development occurs in the thymus, where variable, diversity, and joining T-cell receptor (TCR) gene segments undergo recombination to create diverse TCR specificities and in the process form TRECS as byproducts. An absence of TRECs correlates with a lack of production of thymic emigrant T cells. All infants with SCID fail to generate a diverse repertoire of mature T cells, and consequently have undetectable or very low numbers of TRECs.[6,7] Whether the underlying SCID gene defect prevents

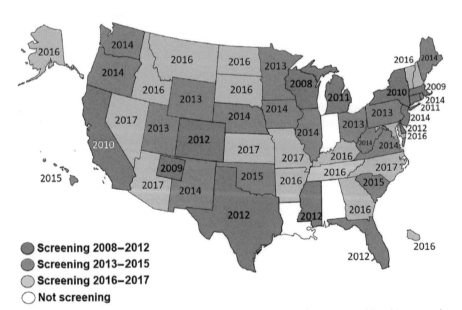

Fig. 1. Map of United States showing the implementation of severe combined immunodeficiency (SCID) newborn screening. Dark shading, 10 state programs and the Navajo Nation with SCID newborn screening contributing to this study; lighter shading, programs with SCID screening, but not part of this study; lighter still, SCID screening pilot programs, plans, or consideration for SCID newborn screening. The year that screening began is indicated. (*Adapted from* Immune Deficiency Foundation (IDF). IDF SCID Newborn Screening Campaign. Available at: http://primaryimmune.org/idf-advocacy-center/idf-scid-newborn-screening-campaign/. Accessed May 26, 2017; with permission.)

the TCR recombination process itself, impairs cytokine-mediated signaling essential for T-cell maturation and activation, or allows the accumulation of toxic purine metabolites such as with adenosine deaminase deficiency (ADA) SCID, all genotypes are characterized by a paucity of TRECs.

HISTORY AND DEFINITIONS

The definition of SCID has evolved over time. Before SCID NBS, children presented with recurrent, severe and opportunistic bacterial, viral, and fungal infections; diarrhea; and in some cases a positive family history, as in the X-linked inheritance pattern with affected males and immunologically healthy unaffected female carriers of the causative mutation.[8] ADA deficiency was also recognized in 1972 as a metabolic cause of SCID that could be diagnosed biochemically.[9] Although originally fatal in early life, SCID became treatable with the establishment of a working immune system through bone marrow transplantation from a healthy HLA-matched donor, first reported in 1968.[10] Genetic mapping and positional cloning of SCID genes, starting in 1993, with identification of the X-linked SCID gene *IL2RG* encoding the common γ-chain of cytokine receptors,[11,12] has now led to discovery of 17 genes that can cause SCID when mutated.[13]

NBS with TRECs has allowed us to identify newborns within weeks of birth, before infection and other complications have led to failure to thrive, pneumonia, and other life-threatening infections. Because newborns with SCID generally seem to be healthy when identified by NBS, the diagnosis must primarily be based on laboratory test resuls.[4] Infants with typical SCID have fewer than 300 autologous T cells/μL, less than 10% of the lower range of normal proliferation to the mitogen phytohemagglutinin, and/or detectable transplacental maternal T-cell engraftment, with most cases having deleterious mutations in recognized SCID genes (**Fig. 2**). Patients with leaky SCID have 300 to 1500 T cells/μL or more, but have a restricted TCR repertoire and lack naïve T cells. Maternal T-cell engraftment is not detected in leaky SCID, but the T cells are functionally impaired and have limited diversity. A subset of infants with leaky SCID have expansion of oligoclonal dysregulated T cells, leading to adenopathy, erythroderma, with cutaneous and intestinal T-cell infiltration, hepatomegaly, eosinophilia, and highly increased IgE levels, features collectively known as Omenn syndrome.[4]

NBS also identifies infants with low TREC numbers who do not have SCID but nonetheless have few T lymphocytes in the peripheral blood, which is termed TCL. Although most of these infants have recognized syndromic conditions, such as DiGeorge syndrome, others have secondary T lymphopenia owing to conditions such as lymphatic losses after cardiothoracic surgery or owing to congenital defects in the intestines; preterm birth alone is associated with TCL in some infants. Other infants have TCL with no apparent underlying cause and are diagnosed with idiopathic TCL, although if followed over time some of these resolve, whereas others are found to have an immune defect.

EPIDEMIOLOGY

The incidence of SCID is approximately 1 in 65,000 births and does not seem to be changing.[14] The presence of some founder mutations for SCID in isolated population groups, such as Navajo and Apache Native Americans and Amish and Mennonites, increases the frequency of SCID, but overall in the United States there is no evidence that incidence is varying by race, ethnicity, or geographic area.[15] In cultures with high degrees of consanguinity, the incidence of autosomal recessive SCID is

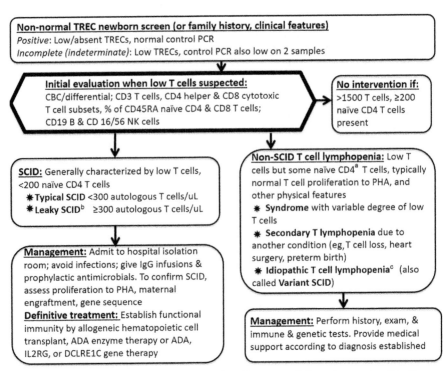

Fig. 2. Evaluation and initial management of T-cell immune defects detected on T-cell receptor excision circle (TREC) newborn screening. Primary immune defects can also be diagnosed based on a history of affected family members or clinical features. [a] Variable can be less than 200 naïve CD4 T cells. [b] Omenn syndrome is a form of leaky severe combined immunodeficiency with rash, eosinophilia, autoreactive, oligoclonal T cells, and a variable CD3 T-cell count, which can be less than 1500. [c] Some infants never leave this group, but some move into this category when other diagnoses are made. These infants need to be followed over time and have different diagnoses. ADA, adenosine deaminase deficiency; CBC, complete blood count; NK, natural killer; PCR, polymerase chain reaction; PHA, phytohemagglutinin. (*Adapted from* Dorsey MJ, Dvorak CC, Cowan MJ, et al. Treatment of infants identified as having severe combined immunodeficiency by means of newborn screening. J Allergy Clin Immunol 2017;139(3):735; with permission.)

substantially higher.[16] In California, which has an ethnically diverse population, infants with clinically significant TCL were identified at a rate of 1 in 15,300 births. Over 6.5 years of screening more than 3 million infants, 50 cases of SCID were found and promptly directed to treatment, which resulted in 96% survival (J. Puck, personal communication, 2018). No cases of typical or early-onset leaky SCID are known to have been missed.

DIFFERENT TYPES OF SEVERE COMBINED IMMUNODEFICIENCY

SCID transplant centers reporting genotypes in infants with SCID detected by NBS show greater proportions of autosomal-recessive gene defects and a lesser proportion of X-linked mutations compared with prior publications. A larger proportion of screened cases are due to defects in *RAG* genes, which often cause leaky SCID and might have been missed or diagnosed later in life without SCID NBS. In contrast with cases reported in the prescreening era, a greater proportion of SCID cases detected by NBS have not been identified with known genes for SCID. Distribution of SCID genotypes in the presence of NBS in 11 SCID NBS programs in the United States is illustrated in **Fig. 3**.

NON–SEVERE COMBINED IMMUNODEFICIENCY CONDITIONS IDENTIFIED BY NEWBORN SCREENING

Non-SCID conditions identified by NBS in California fall into 4 categories: syndromes, secondary T lymphopenia, idiopathic T lymphopenia, and preterm birth (**Box 1**). Since screening was initiated in 2010 in California, our institution has evaluated 32 syndromic infants with non-SCID TCL. These cases included 22 cases of DiGeorge syndrome/22q11.2 deletion or TBX1 intragenic mutation; 4 cases of ataxia telangiectasia, coloboma, heart defect, atresia choanae, retarded growth and development, genital abnormality (CHARGE syndrome), and trisomy-21; 1 case each of Noonan syndrome, Kabuki syndrome, congenital lipomatous overgrowth vascular malformations epidermal nevi and spinal/skeletal anomalies (CLOVES syndrome), Fryns syndrome, and EXTL3 deficiency.[17,18] Those conditions involving absent or dysfunctional thymus such as complete DGS and CHARGE syndrome may require thymus tissue transplant for survival, whereas others with affected immunity in the hematopoietic compartment (eg, RAC2 deficiency) require hematopoietic cell transplantation (HCT). Combined immunodeficiencies associated with intact T-cell development beyond the point of TCR gene recombination in the thymus, including ZAP-70 deficiency and MHC class I and II nonexpression, can have normal numbers of TRECs, even though T-cell function is severely impaired. These conditions may, therefore, not be picked up by SCID NBS. Similarly, ataxia telangiectasia, a combined immunodeficiency, seems to be identified by SCID NBS in about one-half of the known cases.[19]

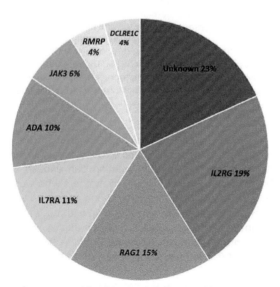

Fig. 3. Distribution of severe combined immunodeficiency (SCID) genotypes reported by 11 SCID NBS programs in the United States with more than 3 million infants screened. Single cases of the following SCID conditions have been identified *BCL11B, CD3D, RAG2,* and *TTC7A*. (*Data from* Kwan A, Abraham RS, Currier R, et al. Newborn screening for severe combined immunodeficiency in 11 screening programs in the United States. JAMA 2014;312 (7):729–38.)

Box 1
Non-SCID conditions identified by SCID NBS in California

Syndromes with variable T-cell deficiency
  DiGeorge/chromosome 22q11.2 deletion[a]
  Trisomy 21
  Ataxia telangiectasia
  CHARGE syndrome[a]
  Diabetic embryopathy[a]
  CLOVES
  EXTL3
  Fryns syndrome
  Nijmegen syndrome[c]
  Noonan syndrome
  RAC2 defect[c]

Secondary T lymphopenia
  Congenital heart disease
  Hydrops
  Gastroschisis
  Chylothorax
  Maternal immunosuppressive medication[b]
  Third-space leakage
  Intestinal atresia
  Meconium ileus
  Teratoma of the thymus

Idiopathic T lymphopenia (no gene defect, few naïve cells, impaired T-cell function)

Preterm birth[d]

Abbreviations: CHARGE, coloboma of the eye, heart defect, atresia choanae, restricted growth and development, genital abnormality, and ear abnormality; CLOVES, congenital, lipomatous, overgrowth, vascular malformations, epidermal nevi and spinal/skeletal anomalies and/or scoliosis; EXTL3, exostosin like glycosyltransferase 3 gene and protein; RAC2, member 2 of Rac subfamily of Rho GTPases; SCID, severe combined immunodeficiency.
  [a] Infants with these conditions have been reported to have undergone thymus transplant.
  [b] Maternal immunosuppressive medication identified include azathioprine and fingolimod.
  [c] Conditions that have been treated with hematopoietic cell transplantation.
  [d] Newborns in this category are typically born at 32 weeks of gestation or earlier.

Causes of secondary TCL include congenital heart disease with vascular leakage, hydrops, chylothorax, gastroschisis, intestinal atresia, and other conditions in which the loss of T cells from the peripheral circulation can exceed production by the thymus. In addition, there were 2 infants born to mothers who were receiving immunosuppressive medications, including fingolimod and azathioprine.

There were 5 infants with idiopathic lymphopenia with no underlying cause identified and some infants who were initially in this category were eventually diagnosed with a syndrome (ataxia telangiectasia). Resolution of idiopathic TCL occurred in 1 infant and 2 continue to be followed with persistence of TCL 1 to 4 years out.[17]

Premature infants and those in the neonatal intensive care unit are a disproportionate source of abnormal TREC results. Kwan and colleagues[20] (2013) reported on the first 2 years of SCID NBS in California. Preterm infants with TCL born at 24 to 27 weeks of gestation with birth weights of 300 to 1200 g had a higher rate of abnormal TREC results than larger, more mature infants. For most infants, subsequent lymphocyte profiles exhibited an improvement in T-cell numbers over time.[20]

EARLY MANAGEMENT AND LABORATORY ASSESSMENT FOR A NEW INFANT WITH SUSPECTED SEVERE COMBINED IMMUNODEFICIENCY

The most important step in the management of suspected SCID is to obtain lymphocyte subset analysis measuring numbers of T, B, and natural killer lymphocytes. Enumeration of naïve and memory T cells (CD45RA/RO) by flow cytometry will provide key information about the infant's ability to generate newly formed T cells and is a key diagnostic test in determining likelihood of SCID or leaky SCID. Individual states in the United States conduct TREC assays differently, and TREC cutoffs for follow-up as well as what type of follow-up occurs also varies. California includes the lymphocyte subset analysis with naïve an memory helper and cytotoxic T cells as an integral part of the NBS process. The accessibility of this second-level testing facilitates early review of results by program immunology consultants, who determine if referral to a primary immunodeficiency center is the next step. Guided by the algorithm in **Fig. 2**, immediate isolation and avoidance of contact with ill persons is advised for infants with suspected SCID. Those infants should not receive live vaccines including the (live-attenuated) rotavirus, and mothers should be advised to suspend breastfeeding until maternal cytomegalovirus (CMV) status is known. This process requires measurement of the mother's serum CMV IgG looking for evidence of prior exposure status. If the mother has evidence of a prior CMV infection, she should not continue to breast feed owing to the risk of transmitting CMV through their breast milk.

Infant care includes directed history with family history including consanguinity, along with careful physical examination focusing on signs of infection, congenital anomalies, rashes, and respiratory status. Confirmation of lymphopenia involves repeating measurement of lymphocyte subsets by flow cytometry including T-cell CD45RA/RO. It has also been recommended to obtain quantitative serum immunoglobulins. In addition, lymphocyte function needs to be evaluated via phytohemagglutinin stimulation. At this point, those infants meeting SCID criteria should start IgG replacement therapy. A chromosome microarray analysis test using single nucleotide polymorphism array hybridization is recommended for infants with cardiac anomalies or features suggestive of DiGeorge or other congenital defects. Further testing includes blood chemistries, albumin, liver function tests, and total bilirubin. Screening tests for infection should include polymerase chain reaction or antigen (not antibody) measurements for adenovirus, CMV, Epstein-Barr virus, hepatitis B, human immunodeficiency virus, herpes simplex virus, and parvovirus B19. Limit blood volumes and do not draw all labs at once to prevent iatrogenic anemia. For prophylaxis, we initiate daily fluconazole and valganciclovir sequentially over the first 2 weeks after the diagnosis and trimethoprim-sulfamethoxazole after 4 weeks of age.

A natural history study of SCID patients treated from 2010 to 2014 identified that active infection before transplantation adversely impacted survival with 80% overall survival for those greater than 3.5 months of age with an active infection at the time of HCT, compared with greater than 90% survival for uninfected infants. Although infants diagnosed via NBS were less likely to have an infection before HCT and presumably less likely to have life-threatening or fatal infections than infants in the prescreening era, 42% still developed infections before HCT.[21] CMV was among the most common infection seen; pneumocystis and candida species infections were seen less commonly in patients diagnosed via NBS or family history. This finding suggests that earlier diagnosis via NBS and early administration of prophylaxis may have prevented these types of infection. It is our practice to monitor CMV through blood or urine polymerase chain reaction every 2 weeks initially, and to continue until after HCT when T-cell immunity is restored. Although previously we would initiate acyclovir prophylaxis we have since discontinued this practice in favor of more CMV-specific prophylaxis with valganciclovir. It is worth noting that bone marrow suppression and oral ulcers are observed side effects in infants. For those who develop these symptoms, the risks and benefits of valganciclovir prophylaxis need to be weighed.

GENETIC WORKUP OF SUSPECTED SEVERE COMBINED IMMUNODEFICIENCY AND T-CELL LYMPHOPENIA

Several options are available for clinical genetic testing when evaluating a newborn suspected of having SCID. The tests most frequently used by clinicians include individual chromosomal microarray analysis, Sanger sequencing (SS), targeted gene panels (TGP), and whole exome sequencing (WES). Whole genome sequencing (WGS) is currently not available in most clinical laboratories, but adoption of this technique is increasing. Chromosomal microarray analysis facilitates the detection of copy number variants, microdeletions, microduplications, and most unbalanced rearrangements of chromosome structure. It may not detect small changes in single genes or balanced translocations. It is a useful genetic test when congenital anomalies suggest a syndrome and has played an essential role in diagnosis of DiGeorge syndrome. SS has been the gold standard in the past for validation of genetic variations, although it is being used less as massively parallel sequencing methods improve.[22] This technique allows for the detection of single nucleotide changes and other small variants with high accuracy. The major disadvantage of SS is that a limited number of candidate genes can be feasibly investigated at any given time. Because there are multiple candidate genes for a given SCID phenotype, SS is less frequently pursued for initial testing than TGP. It is also important to recognize that, in some commercially available diagnostic laboratories, the entire gene is not sequenced, thereby introducing the possibility of missed pathogenic variants. TGPs allow for the investigation of multiple genes at 1 time, typically through next-generation sequencing, including focused analysis of WES. There are several commercially available targeted SCID gene panels currently available. Although TGPs can be designed to detect known intronic variants, they are not typically used for such purposes; therefore, pathogenic intronic variants may be missed.

WES allows for the capture and sequencing of the coding regions of all known genes in the human genome. Because up to 85% of known genetic changes with large effects on disease lie within the exome,[23] this technique represents a relatively high-yield diagnostic modality that may become cost effective, particularly in patients who have no gene identified by TGP approaches. In addition, WES allows for discovery of novel genes where defects may be associated with a given phenotype. Because the coverage of the exon-flanking intronic regions varies, intronic variants can be missed. Furthermore, WES does not typically identify large insertions, deletions, translocations, or inversions. WES is often pursued after a negative TGP in cases of persistent TCL. Finally, WGS provides analysis of the entire genome (both coding and noncoding regions); therefore, interpretation of the data can be extremely time consuming because it relies heavily on clinical expertise. Currently, WGS has limited commercial availability and is cost prohibitive. WES and WGS can identify variants of unknown significance, highlighting the need for functional validation to establish pathogenicity and causal relationship to SCID and TCL.

SPECIAL MANAGEMENT CONSIDERATIONS

Infants with Omenn syndrome owing to hypomorphic mutations in any SCID gene, particularly recombination-activating genes RAG1 and RAG2, require immunosuppression while awaiting hematopoietic stem cell transplantation.

ADA deficiency SCID occurred in one-fifth of cases in the California series. Early complications include neutropenia, which was seen in the majority of California infants with ADA SCID and pulmonary alveolar proteinosis. Pulmonary alveolar proteinosis can lead to respiratory distress and require intubation and ventilatory support in severe cases.[24] These conditions generally resolve once ADA replacement therapy restores adequate levels of the ADA enzyme. This is a reason to institute enzyme therapy promptly for ADA SCID, even while planning more definitive therapy.

Radiation-sensitive SCID includes deficiencies of Artemis, DNA ligase IV, DNA-dependent protein kinase catalytic subunit, Cernunnos-XLF, and nibrin (associated with Nijmegen breakage syndrome). Radiation exposure from radiographs and CT scans should be limited in these patients except when results are necessary to direct management.

Small infants with SCID are susceptible to iatrogenic anemia. Blood draws should be limited to the smallest possible volume to prevent the need for transfusion, which poses risks for infection and allosensitization. Up to 70% of mothers and fathers with infants with SCID experience acute stress disorder and/or depression and symptoms can persist beyond the first year after definitive treatment (M. Dorsey, unpublished data, 2018). The unique psychosocial vulnerability of parents of infants diagnosed with SCID should be recognized and social work interaction is recommended early to identify and support families with a high risk of destabilization of family function.

TREATMENT

HCT is the definitive treatment for SCID when there is a human leukocyte antigen-matched sibling, the ideal donor. Because most patients lack such a donor, alternative donor sources, including unrelated adult donors, haploidentical parents, and cord blood, have been used for allogeneic HCT. The key to successful treatment is to avoid infection in the infant before transplant.[5] Pai and colleagues,[5] in 2014, reported that infants who received transplants before 3.5 months of age had a 5-year survival rate of 94%, similar to infants older than 3.5 months but with no history of infection (90%) or whose infections had fully resolved with treatment by the time of HCT (82%). In contrast, children older than 3.5 months with active infection at the time of HCT and no HLA-matched sibling had the lowest survival rate (50%). Gene therapy for the correction of autologous hematopoietic stem cells through research protocols has been successful for children with ADA and X-linked (IL2RG) SCID. Similarly, gene therapy for Artemis SCID is now available in a clinical trial.

SUMMARY

Advances in SCID NBS over the last 10 years have profoundly improved outcomes of children born with SCID in the United States. Although each state may use different methods for TREC detection and differs in their algorithms for follow-up and tracking of abnormal results, detection of typical and leaky SCID by TREC screening has been universally successful.

REFERENCES

1. IDF SCID Newborn Screening Campaign. Available at: http://primaryimmune.org/idf-advocacy-center/idf-scid-newborn-screening-campaign/. Accessed May 26, 2017.

2. Buckley RH. Molecular defects in human severe combined immunodeficiency and approaches to immune reconstitution. Annu Rev Immunol 2004;22:625–55.
3. Ochs HD, Puck JM. Primary immunodeficiency diseases: a molecular and genetic approach. Oxford (United Kingdom): Oxford University Press; 2013. p. 92.
4. Shearer WT, Dunn E, Notarangelo LD, et al. Establishing diagnostic criteria for severe combined immunodeficiency disease (SCID), leaky SCID, and Omenn syndrome: the primary immune deficiency treatment consortium experience. J Allergy Clin Immunol 2014;133:1092–8.
5. Pai SY, Logan BR, Griffith LM, et al. Transplantation outcomes for severe combined immunodeficiency, 2000–2009. N Engl J Med 2014;371:434–46.
6. Chan K, Puck JM. Development of population-based newborn screening for severe combined immunodeficiency. J Allergy Clin Immunol 2005;115:391–8.
7. Morinishi Y, Imai K, Nakagawa N, et al. Identification of severe combined immunodeficiency by T-cell receptor excision circles quantification using neonatal Guthrie cards. J Pediatr 2009;155:829–33.
8. Hitzig WH, Biro Z, Bosch H, et al. Agammaglobulinemia & alymphocytosis with atrophy of lymphatic tissue. Helv Paediatr Acta 1958;13:551–85.
9. Giblett E, Anderson J, Cohen F, et al. Adenosine-deaminase deficiency in two patients with severely impaired cellular immunity. Lancet 1972;300:1067–9.
10. Gatti R, Meuwissen H, Allen H, et al. Immunological reconstitution of sex-linked lymphopenic immunological deficiency. Lancet 1968;292:366–1369.
11. Noguchi M, Yi H, Rosenblatt HM, et al. Interleukin-2 receptor γ chain mutation results in X-linked severe combined immunodeficiency in humans. Cell 1993;73:47–157.
12. Puck JM, Deschenes SM, Porter JC, et al. The interleukin-2 receptor γ chain maps to Xq13. 1 and is mutated in X-linked severe combined immunodeficiency, SCIDX1. Hum Mol Genet 1993;2:1099–104.
13. Picard C, Gaspar HB, Al-Herz W, et al. International union of immunological societies: 2017 primary immunodeficiency diseases committee report on inborn errors of immunity. J Clin Immunol 2018;38:96–128.
14. Kwan A, Abraham RS, Currier R, et al. Newborn screening for severe combined immunodeficiency in 11 screening programs in the United States. JAMA 2014;312:729–38.
15. Kwan A, Hu D, Song M, et al. Successful newborn screening for SCID in the Navajo Nation. Clin Immunol 2015;158(1):29–34.
16. Al-Mousa H, Al-Dakheel G, Jabr A, et al. High incidence of severe combined immunodeficiency disease in Saudi Arabia detected through combined TREC and next generation sequencing of newborn dried blood spots. Front Immunol 2018;9:1–8.
17. Dorsey MJ, Dvorak CC, Cowan MJ, et al. Treatment of infants identified as having severe combined immunodeficiency by means of newborn screening. J Allergy Clin Immunol 2017;139:733–42.
18. Volpi S, Yamazaki Y, Brauer PM, et al. EXTL3 mutations cause skeletal dysplasia, immune deficiency, and developmental delay. J Exp Med 2017. https://doi.org/10.1084/jem.20161525.
19. Mallott J, Kwan A, Church J, et al. Newborn screening for SCID identifies patients with ataxia telangiectasia. J Clin Immunol 2013;33:540–9.
20. Kwan A, Church JA, Cowan MJ, et al. Newborn screening for severe combined immunodeficiency and T-cell lymphopenia in California: results of the first 2 years. J Allergy Clin Immunol 2013;132:140–50.

21. Heimall J, Logan BR, Cowan MJ, et al. Immune reconstitution and survival of 100 SCID patients post–hematopoietic cell transplant: a PIDTC natural history study. Blood 2017;130(25):2718–27.

22. Mu W, Lu H-M, Chen J, et al. Sanger confirmation is required to achieve optimal sensitivity and specificity in next-generation sequencing panel testing. J Mol Diagn 2016;18:923–32.

23. Choi M, Scholl UI, Ji W, et al. Genetic diagnosis by whole exome capture and massively parallel DNA sequencing. Proc Natl Acad Sci U S A 2009;106: 19096–101.

24. Grunebaum E, Cutz E, Roifman CM. Pulmonary alveolar proteinosis in patients with adenosine deaminase deficiency. J Allergy Clin Immunol 2012;129:1588–93.

Hereditary Autoinflammatory Disorders
Recognition and Treatment

Lori Broderick, MD, PhD

KEYWORDS

- Recurrent fever • Immunodeficiency • Autoinflammation • Innate immunity
- Interleukin-1 • Interferon

KEY POINTS

- Hereditary autoinflammatory diseases are an expanding set of disorders characterized by dysregulation of the innate immune system, largely mediated by interleukin-1β, interferon, and nuclear factor–κB.
- Novel syndromes encompassing autoinflammation and immunodeficiency are driving our understanding of the immune system, and how to best treat patients.
- A translational approach, with careful phenotyping of rare patients combined with basic science research and new therapeutics, continues to enhance our knowledge of autoinflammation and the immune system.

INTRODUCTION

Inflammation is a key physiologic response, leading to the elimination of pathogens and guiding tissue repair processes. For a subset of patients, ineffective inappropriate immune responses take the form of immunodeficiency or hypersensitivity disorders. In rare cases, hyperactive inflammatory responses are the cause of autoinflammatory disease, an expanding set of disorders characterized by dysregulation of the innate immune system.[1,2]

For physicians, the challenge lies in diagnosing these rare conditions. Many of the syndromes have signs and symptoms that mimic allergic and immunodeficiency disorders.[3–5] The constellation of fevers, rashes, and mucosal symptoms in many of the

Conflicts of Interest: Dr L. Broderick is a speaker for Novartis, Inc.

Dr L. Broderick has received grant support from NIH NICHD 5K08HD075830 (current), American Academy of Allergy, Asthma, and Immunology Foundation (current), and previously from the Arthritis National Research Foundation, The Hartwell Foundation, Thrasher Research Fund, and A.P. Giannini Foundation.

Division of Allergy, Immunology and Rheumatology, Department of Pediatrics, University of California, San Diego, 9500 Gilman Drive MC 0760, La Jolla, CA 92093, USA

E-mail address: lbroderick@ucsd.edu

Immunol Allergy Clin N Am 39 (2019) 13–29
https://doi.org/10.1016/j.iac.2018.08.004
0889-8561/19/© 2018 Elsevier Inc. All rights reserved.

disorders suggests that the allergist/immunologist is the appropriate specialist for these patients. The early diagnosis and therapeutic initiation is critical to reducing morbidity and mortality in these rare patients. This review focuses on the expanding spectrum of autoinflammation, the role of the allergist/immunologist in diagnosis, and understanding the available treatments.

OVERVIEW OF AUTOINFLAMMATION

The clinical and molecular features of autoinflammatory diseases have been intimately linked since the late 1990s to early 2000s, using a true translational "bench to bedside" approach, with patient characterization driving ex vivo and in vitro studies revealing molecular cellular dysfunction, and reveal previously unknown immune pathways.[6] The coinciding discovery of the inflammasome as a mechanism of inflammation and mutations in *NLRP3* in patients with cryopyrin-associated periodic syndromes (CAPS), not only laid the groundwork for our understanding of the pathogenic role of the inflammasome in the classic autoinflammatory disorders, but contributed to the development of novel, targeted therapies to treat these patients.[7]

RECOGNITION OF AUTOINFLAMMATION

"It is the history, however, which, from the practical point of view, becomes the chief diagnostic measure," Rackemann[8] published in the *Journal of the American Medical Association* in 1936, establishing precedence for the importance of history in the evaluation of the allergic patient.

Part of the complexity and challenge in diagnosing these systemic immunologic diseases lies in their unusual presentations. The autoinflammatory syndromes may present with several features that are not uncommon to the allergist. Reactions to cold or vaccines, rash, aphthous ulcers, lung disease, failure to thrive, and recurrent fevers of unknown origin, in the absence of malignancy or autoimmune diseases, may all be indications for an allergy/immunology referral (**Table 1**). Although the availability of next-generation sequencing has been important in identifying new disorders, detailed personal and family history can provide crucial information to differentiate between immunologic disorders, including hypersensitivity, immunodeficiency, and autoinflammation.[3–5]

DEFINING QUESTIONS: UNIQUE FEATURES OF AUTOINFLAMMATORY DISORDERS

Specializing physicians and tertiary centers who care for these patients have outlined key questions to allow for a systematic approach in distinguishing autoinflammatory syndromes.[4,5,9] Questions related to the age of onset, and patterns of disease flares (duration, timing of episodes, associated symptoms) can be instrumental in guiding the clinician toward signs of autoinflammation and even to a subset of autoinflammatory disorders. A clear family history can provide insights into disease pathogenesis and inheritability. It is often these clinical features that delineate and define the underlying inflammatory pathway, guiding the clinician toward diagnosis and appropriate therapy.

Too often, the delays in diagnosis result in trials of numerous therapies, from antibiotics to high-dose corticosteroids and biologics. Beyond primary manifestations of disease, the role of these therapies evolving the immunodysregulatory system can provide insight into the immunologic pathways at work. For many autoinflammatory diseases, nontargeted therapies are ineffective, or in some cases may even worsen

Table 1
Features of autoinflammatory diseases common to allergy/immunology

Signs/Symptoms	FCAS	MWS	NOMID	FMF	PAAND	TRAPS	MKD	DIRA	DITRA	NLRC4	PRAAS	SAVI	SIFD	LUBAC	DADA2	APLAID
Urticaria-like rash	■	■	■											■		
Other cutaneous findings			■	■	■	■	■	■	■		■	■	■	■	■	■
Cold-induced symptoms	■									■						
Pulmonary symptoms				■							■	■		■		
Conjunctivitis	■	■	■			■					■					
Recurrent infections							■				■	■	■	■	■	■
Cytopenia											■	■	■	■	■	
Lymphadenopathy/splenomegaly		■	■			■	■				■	■	■			

Abbreviations: APLAID, autoinflammation and PLCγ2-associated antibody deficiency and immune dysregulation; DADA2, deficiency of adenosine deaminase 2; DIRA, deficiency of the IL-1 receptor antagonist; DITRA, deficiency of the interleukin-36 receptor antagonist; FCAS, familial cold autoinflammatory syndrome; FMF, familial Mediterranean fever; LUBAC, linear ubiquitination chain assembly complex; MWS, Muckle-Wells syndrome; MKD, mevalonate kinase deficiency; NOMID, neonatal-onset multisystem inflammatory disorder; PAAND, pyrin-associated autoinflammation with neutrophilic dermatosis; PRAAS, proteasome-associated autoinflammatory syndrome; SAVI, stimulator of interferon genes–associated vasculopathy with onset in infancy; SIFD, sideroblastic anemia, B-cell immunodeficiency, periodic fevers, and developmental delay; TRAPS, TNF-receptor-associated periodic syndrome.
Black boxes indicate symptoms which have been described in each syndrome.

symptoms.[10] Therefore, understanding the biology behind these diseases is emphasized.

CATEGORIES OF AUTOINFLAMMATION

Numerous attempts have been made to classify the autoinflammatory spectrum.[11,12] Although initially linked to neutrophils and the role of interleukin (IL)-1, the family of autoinflammatory diseases has expanded to include inflammatory pathology driven by IL-1, type I interferons, and nuclear factor (NF)-κB.[13] The translational approach to these disorders has been consistent with careful phenotyping of patients, recognition of dysregulation of the innate immune response to foreign and endogenous danger signals leading to enhanced inflammation, and gene identification with orphan disease-driven clinical trials using targeted therapy.

THE INFLAMMASOME AND MECHANISM OF INTERLEUKIN-1 FAMILY DRIVEN INFLAMMATION

The prototypical autoinflammatory diseases are the IL-1–mediated disorders first described with the inflammasome in the late twentieth century.[14–16] Inflammasomes are cytoplasmic sensor complexes that detect exogenous and endogenous danger signals, Exogenous danger signals are conserved microbial signatures, called pathogen-associated molecular patterns, whereas endogenous, metabolic danger signals are damage-associated molecular patterns that are upregulated with cell activation and cell death, including adenosine triphosphate. Many of these danger signals are detected by intracellular pattern recognition sensors, known as the nucleotide-binding oligomerization domainlike receptors (NLRs), which form the core of multimeric protein complexes known as inflammasomes.[14,17] Interaction of component proteins results in activation, and oligomerization, ultimately leading to release of proinflammatory cytokines IL-1 and IL-18, and an inflammatory cascade.

Cryopyrin-Associated Periodic Syndromes (Cryopyrinopathies)

Gain-of-function mutations in *NLRP3* underlie a spectrum of diseases, collectively referred to as CAPS or cryopyrinopathies (**Table 2**).[18–20] Although patients share symptoms of recurrent fever, urticaria-like rash, malaise, headaches, joint pain, and conjunctivitis, clinical features can be used to further delineate where patients fall on the CAPS inflammatory spectrum, although overlap can frequently occur. The mildest form, initially called familial cold urticaria, and later familial cold autoinflammatory syndrome (FCAS), was first described in patients with a cold-induced, autoinflammatory syndrome characterized by short febrile episodes associated with an urticaria-like rash and arthralgias.[21,22] Mutations were subsequently identified in more severely affected patients with Muckle-Wells syndrome (MWS) similarly presenting with episodes of fever, rash, malaise and arthralgias of the large joints. Unlike FCAS, patients may also develop a sensorineural hearing loss in adolescence and have a risk of amyloidosis.[23] The most severe end of the spectrum, NOMID, consists of nearly daily fever, arthralgia, hearing loss, and amyloidosis. Neurosensory symptoms are more severe in NOMID than in MWS, and include chronic aseptic meningitis, headaches, vision impairment, and developmental delay. The development of osseous overgrowth of the epiphyses in the long bones is a defining feature and leads to morbidity and deformity.[24]

Familial Mediterranean Fever

Familial Mediterranean fever (FMF), caused by mutations in *MEFV*, which encodes pyrin, is likely the most well known of the autoinflammatory syndromes.[25] The disease

Table 2
Classic interleukin-1–driven hereditary fever syndromes

	Cryopyrinopathies			FMF	TRAPS	MKD	DIRA
	FCAS	MWS	NOMID				
Gene (inheritance)	NLRP3 (AD)	NLRP3 (AD)	NLRP3 (AD/de novo)	MEFV (AR)	TNFRSF1A (AD)	MVK (AR)	IL1RN (AR)
Age of onset	Infancy	Infancy	Infancy	First decade	Variable	Infancy	Infancy
Duration of attacks	<1 d	2–3 d	Continuous	1–3 d	Days-weeks	3–7 d	Continuous
Cutaneous signs	Urticaria-like rash, cold induced	Urticaria-like rash	Urticaria-like rash	Erysipeloid rash on lower leg, ankle, foot	Migratory rash	Maculopapular rash on trunk and limbs, including palmar/plantar	Neutrophilic pustular rash
Peritoneal symptoms	None	Abdominal pain	Rare	Sterile peritonitis, constipation	Sterile peritonitis	Severe pain, vomiting, diarrhea	Rare
Cardiopulmonary symptoms	None	Rare	Rare	Common	Common	Rare	Rare
Arthropathy	Polyarthralgia	Polyarthralgia, oligoarthritis	Epiphyseal overgrowth, contractures, intermittent or chronic arthritis	Monoarthritis	Arthritis in large joints, arthralgia	Arthralgia, symmetric polyarthritis	Osteopenia with sterile lytic bone lesions

(continued on next page)

Table 2
(continued)

	Cryopyrinopathies			FMF	TRAPS	MKD	DIRA
	FCAS	MWS	NOMID				
Ocular features	Conjunctivitis	Conjunctivitis, episcleritis	Uveitis, conjunctivitis, progressive vision loss	Rare	Conjunctivitis, periorbital edema	Uncommon	Rare
Neurologic features	Headache	Sensorineural deafness	Sensorineural deafness, chronic aseptic meningitis, mental retardation	Rare	Rare	Rare, but ataxia, seizures may be seen with mevalonate aciduria	Not common
Lymphatics/Spleen	Not seen	Rare	Hepatosplenomegaly, adenopathy	Splenomegaly	Splenomegaly	Cervical adenopathy	Splenomegaly
Treatments	IL-1 blockade			Colchicine, IL-1 blockade	Steroids, IL-1 blockade	IL-1 blockade	Anakinra

Abbreviations: AD, autosomal dominant; AR, autosomal recessive; DIRA, deficiency of the IL-1 receptor antagonist; FCAS, familial cold autoinflammatory syndrome; FMF, familial Mediterranean fever; IL, interleukin; MKD, mevalonate kinase deficiency; MWS, Muckle-Wells syndrome; NOMID, neonatal-onset multi-system inflammatory disorder; TRAPS, tumor necrosis factor receptor–associated periodic syndrome.

classically considered to be autosomal recessive in inheritance, but there are increasing reports of patients with only 1 or no identifiable *MEFV* mutations, providing a diagnostic challenge.[26,27] Symptoms of FMF include discrete, short episodes of fever with serositis, synovitis, and occasionally an erysipeloid skin rash localized to the lower extremities. Serologic evaluation demonstrates increased acute-phase reactants. Deposition of reactive amyloid A leads to morbidity and mortality due to nephrotic syndrome and renal failure, but other organ systems also may be affected.[28–30]

Pyrin-Associated Autoinflammation with Neutrophilic Dermatosis

Mutations in pyrin have been linked to a new autosomal dominant syndrome named pyrin-associated autoinflammation with neutrophilic dermatosis (PAAND).[31,32] Patients experienced recurrent episodes of fever, neutrophilic dermatosis, arthralgia, myalgia/myositis and elevated serum acute-phase reactants, beginning in childhood. This disorder has been attributed to 2 mutations to date, both of which appear to mimic a bacterial trigger and subsequently induce inflammasome activation and increased IL-1β production.[31] Differences in serum cytokine protein expression between patients with PAAND and patients with FMF are reflective of the distinct clinical presentations.

Tumor Necrosis Factor Receptor–Associated Periodic Syndrome

Tumor necrosis factor receptor–associated periodic syndrome (TRAPS), previously called Hibernian fever, results from autosomal dominantly inherited or de novo mutations in *TNFRSF1A* with a variable age of onset: from 4 days, through the sixth decade of life, with an average of 3 years.[33] Flares are characterized by episodes of spiking fever lasting days to several weeks, and occur spontaneously or are triggered by a minor illness. Associated symptoms include migrating myalgia, arthralgia of the large joints and wrists, and arthritis. Serosal inflammation in TRAPS, especially of the chest and abdomen, can lead to unnecessary laparoscopy; and the sterile acute peritonitis so closely mimics appendicitis that one-third of patients with TRAPS undergo unnecessary appendectomy.[33] The rash of TRAPS is a centrifugal migratory erythema, although other skin manifestations, including urticaria, have been observed. Patients experience periorbital edema, conjunctivitis, or uveitis. The most worrisome long-term complication of TRAPS is AA amyloidosis, affecting 10% to 20% of untreated patients.[34]

Mevalonate Kinase Deficiency

Mevalonate kinase deficiency (MKD) is a spectrum of 2 diseases: the milder hyperimmunoglobulinemia D and periodic fever syndrome (HIDS) and the more severe mevalonic aciduria (MA). Both result from autosomal recessive mutations in *MVK* gene encoding mevalonate kinase, an enzyme in the cholesterol and isoprenoid synthesis pathway.[35] Enzyme activity is reduced/absent due to mutation effects on protein stability. Defective prenylation leads to increased IL-1β secretion.[36] The febrile episodes in MKD typically last 3 to 7 days, and occur every 2 to 12 weeks, although episodes tend to become less frequent with age. Associated symptoms may include lymphadenopathy, abdominal pain, polyarthralgias, myalgia, oral mucosal ulcers, and a palmar/plantar maculopapular rash, although increasing variability among patients is observed.[37,38] A subset of patients present with neurologic findings including ataxia and seizures; this is more likely to be on the MA end of the spectrum. Febrile episodes in MKD maybe triggered by immunizations prompting an allergy referral for vaccine reactions. Laboratory evaluation shows elevated immunoglobulin (Ig)D and IgA levels, although up to 20% of patients will not have an elevated IgD.[39] Urine studies may show elevated mevalonic acid excretion.[40] Most patients have been described in the Netherlands, with a carrier frequency estimated as high as 1:65.[41] However, the identification of patients from other ethnic backgrounds and variable presentation suggests that variability exists along the disease spectrum, and that modifier genes also may play a role in disease phenotype.[42]

Deficiencies of Receptor Antagonists: Deficiency of the Interleukin-1 Receptor Antagonist and Deficiency of the Interleukin-36 Receptor Antagonist

As a powerful driver of innate immune pathways, the inflammasome has multiple regulatory checkpoints, including receptor antagonists. In the past few years, several groups have identified patients presenting with neutrophilic pustular rashes and systemic inflammation. Autosomal recessive mutations were identified in *IL1RN*, the IL-1 receptor antagonist, and *IL36RN*,[43] encoding the IL-36 receptor antagonist,[44] both key inhibitory molecules in the IL-1 family.

NLRC4-Related Syndromes

Mutations in NLRC4 have been linked to clinically heterogeneous syndromes. De novo, gain-of-function mutations in *NLRC4* were described in patients with recurrent episodes of fever, urticarial rash, enterocolitis, splenomegaly, and macrophage activation syndrome.[45,46] All patients were found to have elevations in IL-1β and IL-18. A third group described a family with similarities to FCAS: cold-induced episodes of fever and urticaria-like.[47] Last, an infant with a NOMID phenotype, with no identifiable mutation in *NLRP3*, was found to have a somatic mutation in *NLRC4*.[48] Further research will reveal whether the differences between these NLRC4-associated phenotypes represents a spectrum of disorders similar to the cryopyrinopathies, or the effect of different mutations in the context of different genomes or gene-environment interactions, as well as guide the most appropriate therapy.

INTERFERON-MEDIATED DISEASES

Interferons modulate innate (autoinflammatory) and adaptive (autoimmune) pathologic immune responses in addition to the cell-intrinsic and antiviral effect.[49] Similar to IL-1β, interferon production and signaling are highly regulated. Despite their well-recognized role as signaling proteins in viral and bacterial infections, and antitumor responses, interferon-related disorders have only recently been implicated in autoinflammatory disease (**Table 3**).

Proteasome-Associated Autoinflammatory Syndrome

Proteasome-associated autoinflammatory syndrome (PRAAS), denotes a group of patients presenting with recurrent fevers beginning in infancy or early childhood, which were accompanied by nodular erythema, rash, and joint contractures. Patients have lipomuscular atrophy and a mixed cellular infiltrate with predominantly myeloid cells in their skin biopsies. The identification of autosomal recessive or compound heterozygous mutations in the proteasome subunit beta type 8 (*PSMB8*) gene suggests that these syndromes exist on the same spectrum, similar to the cryopyrinopathies. Mutations in *PSMB8* affect the proteolytic activity of the proteosome, leading to accumulation of ubiquitinated and oxidized proteins in the cell. Induction of interferon (IFN), by cold, stress or viruses, leads to further accumulation of intracellular proteins and drives the autoinflammatory cycle.[49]

Table 3
Interferon-driven autoinflammatory syndromes

	Proteasome-Associated Autoinflammatory Syndrome (PRAAS)	Stimulator of Interferon Genes–Associated Vasculopathy with Onset in Infancy (SAVI)
Gene (inheritance)	*PSMB8* (AR)	*TMEM173* (AD, de novo)
Age of onset	Infancy	Infancy
Duration of attacks	Chronic inflammation with frequent flares	Continuous
Cutaneous signs	Annular rash, swollen violaceous eyelids, lipodystrophy	Small-vessel vasculopathy with vasculitis and microthrombosis telangiectasias, nailfold capillary tortuosity, worsened with cold exposure
Peritoneal symptoms	Diarrhea, hepatomegaly	Rare
Cardiopulmonary symptoms	Clubbing of fingers and toes noted	Tachypnea, interstitial lung disease
Arthropathy	Joint contractures, muscle atrophy	Myositis and muscle atrophy
Ocular features	Violaceous eyelid swelling	None
Neurologic features	Aseptic meningitis, developmental delays	Rare
Lymph nodes/spleen	Splenomegaly, lymphadenopathy	Hilar/paratracheal lymphadenopathy
Treatments	JAK inhibitors	JAK inhibitors

Abbreviations: AD, autosomal dominant; AR, autosomal recessive; JAK, Janus kinase.

Stimulator of Interferon Genes–Associated Vasculopathy with Onset in Infancy

Stimulator of IFN genes (STING)-associated vasculopathy with onset in infancy (SAVI) is an interferonopathy caused by de novo, gain-of-function mutations in *TMEM173*.[50] *TMEM173* encodes the viral sensor, STING, and SAVI-associated mutations result in constitutive upregulation of IFN-β. Patients present in early infancy with rash or tachypnea, and develop cold-induced, telangiectatic, pustular, or blistering rash on the cheeks, nose, fingers, and toes. Acral vasculitis leads to loss of digits, and vasculitis in the pulmonary vasculature results in interstitial lung disease and mortality.[51,52] Patients may have intermittent low-grade fevers, and develop recurrent infections, specifically skin infections and recurrent pneumonia. Serum evaluation shows elevated C-reactive protein and erythrocyte sedimentation rate, as well as elevated IgG, IgA, and positive autoantibodies.[51,52] Skin biopsy demonstrates small-vessel inflammation with leukocytoclasia. Lung and muscle biopsy show lymphocytic infiltrates in the lung parenchyma and between the muscle fibers, respectively.[50]

AUTOINFLAMMATORY DISEASE WITH FEATURES OF IMMUNODEFICIENCY

As additional patients presented with inflammatory symptoms, novel disorders in which patients present with the seemingly paradoxic phenotypes of autoinflammation and immunodeficiency were described.[53,54] IL-1 and IFN-driven crossover disorders are the consequence of heightened innate immune inflammation; however, clinical observations of hypogammaglobulinemia and B-cell or T-cell immunodeficiency provide insight into the links between adaptive and innate immunity.

Sideroblastic Anemia, B-Cell Immunodeficiency, Periodic Fevers, and Developmental Delay

In 2013, a subset of patients with congenital sideroblastic anemias was found to have associated B immunodeficiency, periodic fevers, and development delay.[55] Seizures, cerebellar atrophy, brittle hair, and sensorineural hearing loss were also described with multiorgan failure and median survival of 48 months. These patients were subsequently found to have bi-allelic mutations in *TRNT1*, encoding an enzyme essential for maturation of transfer RNAs required for protein synthesis.[56] Failure to maintain protein homeostasis results in negative effects on protein clearance and cell survival, leading to release of intracellular mediators from necrotic cells. Patients were also found to have hypogammaglobulinemia and B-cell lymphopenia, whereas T and natural killer cells appear to be low or normal in number.[56–58] Further evaluation has shown that there is an increase in immature B cells, indicating that failure of normal B-cell maturation lies behind the observed lymphopenia.[57]

Linear Ubiquitination Chain Assembly Complex Deficiencies

As described previously, protein homeostasis is necessary for cellular survival and response to stress stimuli. Posttranslational modifications, such as ubiquitination, can further direct immune responses by regulating protein interactions and localization.[59] The linear ubiquitination chain assembly complex (LUBAC) is composed of 3 proteins: the catalytic subunit HOIP, and 2 accessory proteins, HOIL-1 and SHARPIN.[60] Biallelic loss-of-function mutations in 2 of the subunits have been described, resulting in dysregulation of NF-κB–directed immune pathways. HOIL-1[53] and HOIP[61] deficiencies are characterized by early-onset fevers, recurrent viral and bacterial infections, lymphadenopathy, and failure to thrive. Mutations destabilize the LUBAC structure, with persistent activation of monocytes resulting in increased IL-1, IL-6, and IL-8. Chronic inflammation in a subset of patients may lead to amylopectinlike deposits in muscle. HOIL-1 deficiency demonstrates reduced numbers of memory B cells, whereas HOIP showed hypogammaglobulinemia and nonprotective antibody responses to encapsulated bacteria, including *Streptococcus pneumoniae* and *Haemophilus influenzae*. HOIP deficiency has also been reported to have a prominent T-cell lymphopenia, suggesting that, similar to inborn errors of NF-κB,[62] germline mutations in LUBAC pathway proteins, may be a cause of primary T-cell deficiencies.

Deficiency of Adenosine Deaminase 2

Patients with deficiency of adenosine deaminase 2 (DADA2) have autosomal recessively inherited mutations in *CERC1*, encoding adenosine deaminase 2 (ADA2).[63,64] Patients demonstrate fever, livedo racemosa, urticarial papules, and early-onset lacunar strokes.[63,64] Patients with DADA2 may exhibit features of mild immunodeficiency, including pancytopenia or leukocytopenia, and hypogammaglobulinemia. Skin biopsies demonstrate an excess of neutrophils and macrophages.[64] Unlike ADA1 deficiency, disease in DADA2 is not due to the toxic accumulation of adenosine and deoxyadenosine. Rather, ADA2 is thought to be important in normal endothelial development and in the differentiation of anti-inflammatory macrophages, resulting in skewing toward M1 inflammatory macrophages, and increased IL-1β, tumor necrosis factor (TNF) and interferons. Patients with DADA2 have reduced memory B cells and consistently low IgM despite a normal T-cell compartment, consistent with a role in B-cell maturation. In addition, a small percentage of patients may present with neutropenia, suggesting a role for ADA2 in neutrophil development.[65]

Autoinflammation and PLCγ2-Associated Antibody Deficiency and Immune Dysregulation

Dominantly inherited mutations resulting in enzymatic gain-of-function of phospholipase Cγ *(PLCG2)* were identified in 2 patients with recurrent, neutrophilic and eosinophilic, blistering skin lesions, interstitial pneumonitis with bronchiolitis, arthralgia, ocular inflammation, and enterocolitis.[54] Cellulitis and recurrent sinopulmonary infections with an absence of class-switched memory B cells were also described. Despite the common gene, autoinflammation and PLCγ2-associated antibody deficiency and immune dysregulation does not have the cold-induced urticarial symptoms seen in patients with phospholipase Cγ2-associated antibody deficiency and immune dysregulation, which are associated with antibody deficiency, recurrent infections, allergic disease, and autoimmune disease.[66]

CLINICAL EVALUATION OF AUTOINFLAMMATION

The autoinflammatory disorders have numerous defining similarities: recurrent or acute-on-chronic episodes of tissue-specific inflammation, a paucity of autoantibodies and antigen-specific T cells, and symptoms driven by innate immune pathways. Beyond history, several evaluations can be informative in distinguishing among the different disorders, and identifying the underlying pathway.

Serologic Evaluation

The molecular hallmarks of autoinflammatory diseases are evident in the peripheral blood and align with disease pathophysiology. For IL-1–driven disorders, patients exhibit a neutrophilic leukocytosis during inflammatory episodes, whereas for the interferonopathies, cytopenias are more often seen. Serum inflammatory markers are invariably elevated during febrile episodes; however, evaluation of acute/subclinical and chronic inflammation, that is, high-sensitivity C-reactive protein or serum amyloid A, can aid in measuring response to therapy. Evaluation of quantitative immunoglobulins, vaccine responses, and lymphocyte subsets and function can be helpful in distinguishing between autoinflammation and immunodeficiency. However, the newer disease classifications, such as DADA2, have an increasing appreciation of associated immunodeficiency. Compounded by delays in diagnosis, questions remain of whether the observed laboratory abnormalities are an intrinsic defect or a consequence of perturbations induced by chronic inflammation.

Genetic Evaluation in Autoinflammatory Diseases

Genetic determination of disease-causing genes has long been established as a key part of the clinical evaluation of patients with autoinflammatory disorders. The identification of a known disease-causing variant can confirm diagnosis and expedite therapy. Beyond providing an end to the diagnostic journey, genetic confirmation can also assist in the evaluation of extended family members. In addition, a genetic diagnosis aids in defining prognosis. Some variants have known genotype–phenotype correlations, whereas others have different prognostic outcomes depending on the overall genetic context or ethnic background of the patient.[67–71]

As increasing numbers of patients are sequenced, clinicians are recognizing the limitations, largely related to the lack of an identifiable disease-causing mutation and the unclear pathogenicity of certain variants. Somatic mosaicism has been offered as an explanation for most of these so-called mutation-negative patients, with the findings that mutations in as few as 4.2% of cells can lead to classic disease.[72] Early results in NOMID and TRAPS somatic cases suggest that typical therapy leads to improvement or resolution of symptoms and normalization of serum inflammatory markers. It is likely similar findings will be described in other autosomal dominant autoinflammatory disorders.

Low-penetrance variants have been described in several classic autoinflammatory diseases, in unaffected family members, and at low frequencies in normal control populations, which raises questions about the significance of these findings. These variants may function as susceptibility alleles, making the carrier more likely to develop an inflammatory phenotype.[73] Studies of patients with common low-penetrance variants in NLRP3,[74] and TNFRSF1A,[75] have demonstrated that disease may present with clinical symptoms distinct from the classic descriptions. Some patients will have spontaneous resolution of symptoms or a milder course, others may still respond to traditional therapies.[74,75] For the clinician, the ongoing challenge will be in determining the clinical relevance of such variants. Beyond genetics, the field of autoinflammation has largely been established by careful phenotypic analysis of patients, making detailed history taking and recall of episodes invaluable.

TREATMENT

A hallmark of the close link between autoinflammatory disorders and translational research has been the identification of targeted therapy.[6] Methodical, small-scale studies, repurposing of available biologics, in conjunction with orphan disease approval has led to Food and Drug Administration (FDA) approvals for specific therapies for autoinflammatory diseases.[76–79]

Cytokine-Targeted Therapy

The increasing availability in biologics coincided with the initial descriptions of autoinflammatory patients, and generated key in vivo confirmation of the innate inflammatory pathways affected. Initial small series and open-label studies of anakinra (recombinant IL-1-receptor antagonist) demonstrated dramatic reductions in serologic inflammatory markers and disease manifestations across CAPS phenotypes.[76–79] It has been used to treat several other IL-1–driven disorders, including colchicine-resistant FMF, TRAPS, HIDS, and deficiency of the interleukin-1 receptor antagonist and deficiency of the interleukin-36 receptor antagonist.[44,80–82] Two other novel IL-1–targeting therapies, rilonacept and canakinumab, are approved for the treatment of FCAS and MWS, and canakinumab received FDA approval for FMF, TRAPS, and HIDS. All 3 IL-1–targeting drugs have similar safety profiles, with an increased risk of nonopportunistic bacterial infections.

Small Molecule Therapy

Although biologic therapy of autoinflammatory diseases has been instrumental in reducing inflammation, the injectable delivery methods, cost, and patient preference for orally administered drugs has led to a search for small molecule inhibitors of autoinflammation. Treatment with daily oral colchicine can prevent acute inflammatory attacks in FMF, as well as the development of amyloidosis. However, a subset of patients fails to respond to colchicine, or cannot tolerate the gastrointestinal adverse effects, and may benefit from IL-1 blockade. New understanding of the molecular structure of the inflammasome has driven investigations of inflammasome-targeting drugs.[83–85]

For PRAAS, blockade with anakinra, anti-TNF therapy, or inhibitors of the IL-6 receptor led to partial therapeutic success. However, further delineation of the role of the immunoproteosome, combined with the prominent IFN signature, suggested that targeting IFN would provide greater success.[50,52] For the monogenic interferono-pathies, symptoms improved in patients under therapy with the Janus kinase inhibitors. However, the identification of new patients continues to provide therapeutic challenges. Patients are increasingly described with incomplete response to biologics, raising questions of how cytokine modulation affects the innate inflammatory cascade. In addition, the phenotypic variability seen, especially among different age groups, suggests that time, chronic inflammation, and/or epigenetic changes may play a role in the disease and treatment process.

SUMMARY

Over the past several decades, the autoinflammatory disease category has rapidly expanded, with nearly 30 monogenic autoinflammatory disorders described. New case descriptions of patients and presentations has helped to solidify our understanding of the autoinflammatory disorders, but also highlighted the variability between individual patients. Early recognition remains critical to the identification of these patients, and is supported by increasing use of next-generation sequencing in clinical centers. Together with the preclinical advances in understanding underlying inflammatory pathways, physicians and researchers can continue to lead the translational study and treatment of these patients.

REFERENCES

1. Masters SL, Simon A, Aksentijevich I, et al. Horror autoinflammaticus: the molecular pathophysiology of autoinflammatory disease (*). Annu Rev Immunol 2009; 27:621–68.
2. Stoffels M, Kastner DL. Old dogs, new tricks: monogenic autoinflammatory disease unleashed. Annu Rev Genomics Hum Genet 2016;17:245–72.
3. Broderick L. Recurrent fevers for the pediatric immunologist: it's not all immunodeficiency. Curr Allergy Asthma Rep 2016;16(1):2.
4. Kallinich T, Gattorno M, Grattan CE, et al. Unexplained recurrent fever: when is autoinflammation the explanation? Allergy 2013;68(3):285–96.
5. Long SS. Distinguishing among prolonged, recurrent, and periodic fever syndromes: approach of a pediatric infectious diseases subspecialist. Pediatr Clin North Am 2005;52(3):811–35, vii.
6. Holzinger D, Kessel C, Omenetti A, et al. From bench to bedside and back again: translational research in autoinflammation. Nat Rev Rheumatol 2015;11(10): 573–85.
7. Broderick L, De Nardo D, Franklin BS, et al. The inflammasomes and autoinflammatory syndromes. Annu Rev Pathol 2015;10:395–424.
8. Rackemann FM. History taking in allergic diseases. JAMA 1936;106(12):976–9.
9. Gattorno M, Sormani MP, D'Osualdo A, et al. A diagnostic score for molecular analysis of hereditary autoinflammatory syndromes with periodic fever in children. Arthritis Rheum 2008;58(6):1823–32.
10. Nedjai B, Hitman GA, Quillinan N, et al. Proinflammatory action of the antiinflammatory drug infliximab in tumor necrosis factor receptor-associated periodic syndrome. Arthritis Rheum 2009;60(2):619–25.
11. Pathak S, McDermott MF, Savic S. Autoinflammatory diseases: update on classification diagnosis and management. J Clin Pathol 2017;70(1):1–8.
12. Russo RA, Brogan PA. Monogenic autoinflammatory diseases. Rheumatology (Oxford) 2014;53(11):1927–39.

13. de Jesus AA, Canna SW, Liu Y, et al. Molecular mechanisms in genetically defined autoinflammatory diseases: disorders of amplified danger signaling. Annu Rev Immunol 2015;33:823–74.
14. Martinon F, Burns K, Tschopp J. The inflammasome: a molecular platform triggering activation of inflammatory caspases and processing of proIL-beta. Mol Cell 2002;10(2):417–26.
15. Agostini L, Martinon F, Burns K, et al. NALP3 forms an IL-1beta-processing inflammasome with increased activity in Muckle-Wells autoinflammatory disorder. Immunity 2004;20(3):319–25.
16. Ogura Y, Sutterwala FS, Flavell RA. The inflammasome: first line of the immune response to cell stress. Cell 2006;126(4):659–62.
17. Srinivasula SM, Poyet JL, Razmara M, et al. The PYRIN-CARD protein ASC is an activating adaptor for caspase-1. J Biol Chem 2002;277(24):21119–22.
18. Cuisset L, Drenth JP, Berthelot JM, et al. Genetic linkage of the Muckle-Wells syndrome to chromosome 1q44. Am J Hum Genet 1999;65(4):1054–9.
19. Hoffman HM, Mueller JL, Broide DH, et al. Mutation of a new gene encoding a putative pyrin-like protein causes familial cold autoinflammatory syndrome and Muckle-Wells syndrome. Nat Genet 2001;29(3):301–5.
20. Aksentijevich I, Nowak M, Mallah M, et al. De novo CIAS1 mutations, cytokine activation, and evidence for genetic heterogeneity in patients with neonatal-onset multisystem inflammatory disease (NOMID): a new member of the expanding family of pyrin-associated autoinflammatory diseases. Arthritis Rheum 2002; 46(12):3340–8.
21. Hoffman HM, Wanderer AA, Broide DH. Familial cold autoinflammatory syndrome: phenotype and genotype of an autosomal dominant periodic fever. J Allergy Clin Immunol 2001;108(4):615–20.
22. Hoffman HM, Wright FA, Broide DH, et al. Identification of a locus on chromosome 1q44 for familial cold urticaria. Am J Hum Genet 2000;66(5):1693–8.
23. Muckle TJ, Well SM. Urticaria, deafness, and amyloidosis: a new heredo-familial syndrome. Q J Med 1962;31:235–48.
24. Hashkes PJ, Lovell DJ. Recognition of infantile-onset multisystem inflammatory disease as a unique entity. J Pediatr 1997;130(4):513–5.
25. Ancient missense mutations in a new member of the RoRet gene family are likely to cause familial Mediterranean fever. The International FMF Consortium. Cell 1997;90(4):797–807.
26. Booth DR, Gillmore JD, Lachmann HJ, et al. The genetic basis of autosomal dominant familial Mediterranean fever. Q J Med 2000;93(4):217–21.
27. Booty MG, Chae JJ, Masters SL, et al. Familial Mediterranean fever with a single MEFV mutation: where is the second hit? Arthritis Rheum 2009;60(6):1851–61.
28. Ben-Chetrit E. Familial Mediterranean fever (FMF) and renal AA amyloidosis—phenotype-genotype correlation, treatment and prognosis. J Nephrol 2003; 16(3):431–4.
29. Ben-Chetrit E, Backenroth R. Amyloidosis induced, end stage renal disease in patients with familial Mediterranean fever is highly associated with point mutations in the MEFV gene. Ann Rheum Dis 2001;60(2):146–9.
30. Zemer D, Pras M, Sohar E, et al. Colchicine in the prevention and treatment of the amyloidosis of familial Mediterranean fever. N Engl J Med 1986;314(16): 1001–5.
31. Masters SL, Lagou V, Jeru I, et al. Familial autoinflammation with neutrophilic dermatosis reveals a regulatory mechanism of pyrin activation. Sci Transl Med 2016;8(332):332ra345.

32. Moghaddas F, Llamas R, De Nardo D, et al. A novel pyrin-associated autoinflammation with neutrophilic dermatosis mutation further defines 14-3-3 binding of pyrin and distinction to Familial Mediterranean Fever. Ann Rheum Dis 2017; 76(12):2085–94.

33. McDermott EM, Smillie DM, Powell RJ. Clinical spectrum of familial Hibernian fever: a 14-year follow-up study of the index case and extended family. Mayo Clin Proc 1997;72(9):806–17.

34. Obici L, Merlini G. Amyloidosis in autoinflammatory syndromes. Autoimmun Rev 2012;12(1):14–7.

35. van der Meer JW, Vossen JM, Radl J, et al. Hyperimmunoglobulinaemia D and periodic fever: a new syndrome. Lancet 1984;1(8386):1087–90.

36. Mulders-Manders CM, Simon A. Hyper-IgD syndrome/mevalonate kinase deficiency: what is new? Semin Immunopathol 2015;37(4):371–6.

37. Cush JJ. Autoinflammatory syndromes. Dermatol Clin 2013;31(3):471–80.

38. Favier LA, Schulert GS. Mevalonate kinase deficiency: current perspectives. Appl Clin Genet 2016;9:101–10.

39. Zhang S. Natural history of mevalonate kinase deficiency: a literature review. Pediatr Rheumatol Online J 2016;14(1):30.

40. Jeyaratnam J, Ter Haar NM, de Sain-van der Velden MG, et al. Diagnostic value of urinary mevalonic acid excretion in patients with a clinical suspicion of Mevalonate Kinase Deficiency (MKD). JIMD Rep 2016;27:33–8.

41. Houten SM, van Woerden CS, Wijburg FA, et al. Carrier frequency of the V377I (1129G>A) MVK mutation, associated with Hyper-IgD and periodic fever syndrome, in the Netherlands. Eur J Hum Genet 2003;11(2):196–200.

42. Moura R, Tricarico PM, Campos Coelho AV, et al. GRID2 a novel gene possibly associated with mevalonate kinase deficiency. Rheumatol Int 2015;35(4):657–9.

43. Aksentijevich I, Masters SL, Ferguson PJ, et al. An autoinflammatory disease with deficiency of the interleukin-1-receptor antagonist. N Engl J Med 2009;360(23): 2426–37.

44. Rossi-Semerano L, Piram M, Chiaverini C, et al. First clinical description of an infant with interleukin-36-receptor antagonist deficiency successfully treated with anakinra. Pediatrics 2013;132(4):e1043–7.

45. Canna SW, de Jesus AA, Gouni S, et al. An activating NLRC4 inflammasome mutation causes autoinflammation with recurrent macrophage activation syndrome. Nat Genet 2014;46(10):1140–6.

46. Volker-Touw CM, de Koning HD, Giltay JC, et al. Erythematous nodes, urticarial rash and arthralgias in a large pedigree with NLRC4-related autoinflammatory disease, expansion of the phenotype. Br J Dermatol 2017;176(1):244–8.

47. Kitamura A, Sasaki Y, Abe T, et al. An inherited mutation in NLRC4 causes autoinflammation in human and mice. J Exp Med 2014;211(12):2385–96.

48. Kawasaki Y, Oda H, Ito J, et al. Identification of a high-frequency somatic NLRC4 mutation as a cause of autoinflammation by pluripotent cell-based phenotype dissection. Arthritis Rheumatol 2017;69(2):447–59.

49. Schindler C, Levy DE, Decker T. JAK-STAT signaling: from interferons to cytokines. J Biol Chem 2007;282(28):20059–63.

50. Liu Y, Ramot Y, Torrelo A, et al. Mutations in proteasome subunit beta type 8 cause chronic atypical neutrophilic dermatosis with lipodystrophy and elevated temperature with evidence of genetic and phenotypic heterogeneity. Arthritis Rheum 2012;64(3):895–907.

51. Clarke SL, Pellowe EJ, de Jesus AA, et al. Interstitial lung disease caused by STING-associated vasculopathy with onset in infancy. Am J Respir Crit Care Med 2016;194(5):639–42.
52. Liu Y, Jesus AA, Marrero B, et al. Activated STING in a vascular and pulmonary syndrome. N Engl J Med 2014;371(6):507–18.
53. Boisson B, Laplantine E, Prando C, et al. Immunodeficiency, autoinflammation and amylopectinosis in humans with inherited HOIL-1 and LUBAC deficiency. Nat Immunol 2012;13(12):1178–86.
54. Zhou Q, Lee GS, Brady J, et al. A hypermorphic missense mutation in PLCG2, encoding phospholipase Cgamma2, causes a dominantly inherited autoinflammatory disease with immunodeficiency. Am J Hum Genet 2012;91(4):713–20.
55. Wiseman DH, May A, Jolles S, et al. A novel syndrome of congenital sideroblastic anemia, B-cell immunodeficiency, periodic fevers, and developmental delay (SIFD). Blood 2013;122(1):112–23.
56. Chakraborty PK, Schmitz-Abe K, Kennedy EK, et al. Mutations in TRNT1 cause congenital sideroblastic anemia with immunodeficiency, fevers, and developmental delay (SIFD). Blood 2014;124(18):2867–71.
57. Giannelou A, Wang H, Zhou Q, et al. Aberrant tRNA processing causes an autoinflammatory syndrome responsive to TNF inhibitors. Ann Rheum Dis 2018;77(4): 612–9.
58. Lougaris V, Chou J, Baronio M, et al. Novel biallelic TRNT1 mutations resulting in sideroblastic anemia, combined B and T cell defects, hypogammaglobulinemia, recurrent infections, hypertrophic cardiomyopathy and developmental delay. Clin Immunol 2018;188:20–2.
59. Corn JE, Vucic D. Ubiquitin in inflammation: the right linkage makes all the difference. Nat Struct Mol Biol 2014;21(4):297–300.
60. Aksentijevich I, Zhou Q. NF-kappaB pathway in autoinflammatory diseases: dysregulation of protein modifications by ubiquitin defines a new category of autoinflammatory diseases. Front Immunol 2017;8:399.
61. Boisson B, Laplantine E, Dobbs K, et al. Human HOIP and LUBAC deficiency underlies autoinflammation, immunodeficiency, amylopectinosis, and lymphangiectasia. J Exp Med 2015;212(6):939–51.
62. Doffinger R, Smahi A, Bessia C, et al. X-linked anhidrotic ectodermal dysplasia with immunodeficiency is caused by impaired NF-kappaB signaling. Nat Genet 2001;27(3):277–85.
63. Navon Elkan P, Pierce SB, Segel R, et al. Mutant adenosine deaminase 2 in a polyarteritis nodosa vasculopathy. N Engl J Med 2014;370(10):921–31.
64. Zhou Q, Yang D, Ombrello AK, et al. Early-onset stroke and vasculopathy associated with mutations in ADA2. N Engl J Med 2014;370(10):911–20.
65. Caorsi R, Penco F, Grossi A, et al. ADA2 deficiency (DADA2) as an unrecognised cause of early onset polyarteritis nodosa and stroke: a multicentre national study. Ann Rheum Dis 2017;76(10):1648–56.
66. Milner JD. PLAID: a syndrome of complex patterns of disease and unique phenotypes. J Clin Immunol 2015;35(6):527–30.
67. Aksentijevich I, Putnam CD, Remmers EF, et al. The clinical continuum of cryopyrinopathies: novel CIAS1 mutations in North American patients and a new cryopyrin model. Arthritis Rheum 2007;56(4):1273–85.
68. Aksentijevich I, Galon J, Soares M, et al. The tumor-necrosis-factor receptor-associated periodic syndrome: new mutations in TNFRSF1A, ancestral origins, genotype-phenotype studies, and evidence for further genetic heterogeneity of periodic fevers. Am J Hum Genet 2001;69(2):301–14.

69. Cazeneuve C, Sarkisian T, Pecheux C, et al. MEFV-Gene analysis in Armenian patients with Familial Mediterranean fever: diagnostic value and unfavorable renal prognosis of the M694V homozygous genotype-genetic and therapeutic implications. Am J Hum Genet 1999;65(1):88–97.
70. Kone Paut I, Dubuc M, Sportouch J, et al. Phenotype-genotype correlation in 91 patients with familial Mediterranean fever reveals a high frequency of cutaneomucous features. Rheumatology (Oxford) 2000;39(11):1275–9.
71. Mandey SH, Schneiders MS, Koster J, et al. Mutational spectrum and genotype-phenotype correlations in mevalonate kinase deficiency. Hum Mutat 2006;27(8): 796–802.
72. Tanaka N, Izawa K, Saito MK, et al. High incidence of NLRP3 somatic mosaicism in patients with chronic infantile neurologic, cutaneous, articular syndrome: results of an International Multicenter Collaborative Study. Arthritis Rheum 2011; 63(11):3625–32.
73. Shinar Y, Obici L, Aksentijevich I, et al. Guidelines for the genetic diagnosis of hereditary recurrent fevers. Ann Rheum Dis 2012;71(10):1599–605.
74. Verma D, Lerm M, Blomgran Julinder R, et al. Gene polymorphisms in the NALP3 inflammasome are associated with interleukin-1 production and severe inflammation: relation to common inflammatory diseases? Arthritis Rheum 2008;58(3): 888–94.
75. Ruiz-Ortiz E, Iglesias E, Soriano A, et al. Disease phenotype and outcome depending on the age at disease onset in patients carrying the R92Q low-penetrance variant in TNFRSF1A gene. Front Immunol 2017;8:299.
76. Goldbach-Mansky R, Dailey NJ, Canna SW, et al. Neonatal-onset multisystem inflammatory disease responsive to interleukin-1beta inhibition. N Engl J Med 2006; 355(6):581–92.
77. Hawkins PN, Lachmann HJ, McDermott MF. Interleukin-1-receptor antagonist in the Muckle-Wells syndrome. N Engl J Med 2003;348(25):2583–4.
78. Hoffman HM, Rosengren S, Boyle DL, et al. Prevention of cold-associated acute inflammation in familial cold autoinflammatory syndrome by interleukin-1 receptor antagonist. Lancet 2004;364(9447):1779–85.
79. Hoffman HM, Throne ML, Amar NJ, et al. Efficacy and safety of rilonacept (interleukin-1 Trap) in patients with cryopyrin-associated periodic syndromes: results from two sequential placebo-controlled studies. Arthritis Rheum 2008;58(8): 2443–52.
80. Cailliez M, Garaix F, Rousset-Rouviere C, et al. Anakinra is safe and effective in controlling hyperimmunoglobulinaemia D syndrome-associated febrile crisis. J Inherit Metab Dis 2006;29(6):763.
81. Gattorno M, Pelagatti MA, Meini A, et al. Persistent efficacy of anakinra in patients with tumor necrosis factor receptor-associated periodic syndrome. Arthritis Rheum 2008;58(5):1516–20.
82. Mitroulis I, Papadopoulos VP, Konstantinidis T, et al. Anakinra suppresses familial Mediterranean fever crises in a colchicine-resistant patient. Neth J Med 2008; 66(11):489–91.
83. Coll RC, Robertson AA, Chae JJ, et al. A small-molecule inhibitor of the NLRP3 inflammasome for the treatment of inflammatory diseases. Nat Med 2015;21(3): 248–55.
84. Garcia-Carbonero R, Carnero A, Paz-Ares L. Inhibition of HSP90 molecular chaperones: moving into the clinic. Lancet Oncol 2013;14(9):e358–69.
85. Lamkanfi M, Malireddi RK, Kanneganti TD. Fungal zymosan and mannan activate the cryopyrin inflammasome. J Biol Chem 2009;284(31):20574–81.

Secondary Hypogammaglobulinemia

An Increasingly Recognized Complication of Treatment with Immunomodulators and After Solid Organ Transplantation

Blanka Kaplan, MD*, Vincent R. Bonagura, MD

KEYWORDS

- Secondary immunodeficiency • Hypogammaglobulinemia • Antibody deficiency
- Immunosuppressive therapy • Immunosuppressive biological therapies
- Hematologic malignancy • Infections • Rituximab

KEY POINTS

- Secondary hypogammaglobulinemia is an increasingly common development in patients treated with immunosuppressive therapy.
- Screening for an underlying immunodeficiency is crucial in people with a history of recurrent, severe, or unusual infections or hematologic malignancies and before transplantation and starting immunomodulatory agents, including biologics.
- Preexistent primary or secondary immunodeficiency is exponentially magnified by immunosuppressive therapy, which can lead to reactivation and acceleration of latent, residual, and opportunistic infections.
- Antibody deficiency is characterized by decreased serum immunoglobulin levels in combination with the inability to mount primary and anamnestic protective antibody responses to vaccinations and infectious antigens.
- Management of secondary hypogammaglobulinemia includes screening for infections before starting immunomodulatory agents as indicated, early vaccination, antiinfective prophylaxis, and replacement immunoglobulin when indicated.

Disclosure Statement: No disclosures (B. Kaplan). Primary Immunodeficiency Disease Advisory Board: CSL-Behring; lecturer on primary immunodeficiency disease: Shire; LINK Advisory Board: Grifols (V.R. Bonagura).
Division of Allergy and Immunology, Donald and Barbara Zucker School of Medicine at Hofstra/Northwell, Steven and Alexandra Cohen Medical Center of New York, 865 Northern Boulevard, Suite 101, Great Neck, NY 11021, USA
* Corresponding author.
E-mail address: bkaplan@northwell.edu

INTRODUCTION

Primary immunodeficiency disorders (PIDDs), defined as inherited conditions that impair the function of the immune system, are distinct from secondary immunodeficiencies (SIDs), which can occur as a consequence of underlying illness, immunosuppressive treatment, and environmental and personal factors. SIDs result from altered immune system function in association with immunosuppressive therapies, malnutrition, infiltrative diseases or malignancies, infectious diseases, protein-losing disorders, structural abnormalities or surgery, certain hereditary disorders, extremes of age, harsh climates, isolation, extreme stress, sleep deprivation, radiation, and idiosyncratic drug-induced adverse effects.[1,2] SIDs are more prevalent than PIDD and are frequently unrecognized by clinicians.

Multiple medications in therapeutic doses can cause hypogammaglobulinemia. Decreased serum immunoglobulin A (IgA) can be caused by various anticonvulsant[3] and psychotropic agents, such as phenytoin, carbamazepine, valproic acid, chlorpromazine,[4] lamotrigine, and zonisamide. There are also reports of lamotrigine and carbamazepine causing decreases in total immunoglobulin G (IgG) and IgG subclasses[5] and a common variable immunodeficiency–like disease.[6,7]

Immunosuppressive therapies (ISTs) are indispensable for treating autoimmune, connective tissue, and malignant diseases and before and after hematopoietic stem cell (HSC) and solid organ transplantation. They are used to induce or maintain clinical remission, to decrease flares, and as steroid-sparing agents. In HSC transplantation, medical ISTs are used for the prevention and treatment of graft-versus-host disease. As the use of immunomodulatory drugs, including biologics, continues to increase, clinicians should be aware of their potential adverse reactions. These reactions include significant effects on innate, cellular, and humoral immunity that in turn can lead to severe, even fatal infections and autoimmune and lymphoproliferative diseases.

Medication-induced immunosuppression can be especially detrimental in patients with underlying immunodeficiency diseases, both primary and secondary. Many immunodeficient patients have a higher risk for developing autoimmunity and malignancy; however, more than 50% of patients with PIDD are not diagnosed until 25 years of age.[8] Consequently, treatment of autoimmunity and malignancy with IST without recognizing the underlying PIDD can put these patients at higher risk for complications. Likewise, hypogammaglobinemia secondary to hematologic malignancy is likely to be aggravated by IST. Hence, screening for preexistent immunodeficiency is crucial to decrease infectious complications of medication-induced immunosuppression. This article reviews immunosuppressive medications that commonly cause hypogammaglobulinemia.

NONBIOLOGICAL IMMUNOSUPPRESSIVE DRUGS THAT CAUSE HYPOGAMMAGLOBULINEMIA

Many of the traditional (nonbiological) immunosuppressive medications are used for the treatment of various autoimmune, malignant, and transplant rejection. Glucocorticoids,[9–11] sulfasalazine, gold, mycophenolate mofetil, methotrexate, azathioprine, and alkylating agents affect various pathways of innate and acquired immunity and can cause cytopenias, lymphocyte dysfunction and decrease immunoglobulin production (**Table 1**). Combining immunosuppressive medications leads to more frequent and severe hypogammaglobulinemia.[12,13] Immunosuppression can be complicated by an increased risk and severity of bacterial, viral, fungal, and protozoan infections, including opportunistic.

Table 1
Immunosuppressive (nonbiological) drugs that cause hypogammaglobulinemia

	Use	Mechanism of Action	Adverse Effects on Immune Cells and Immunoglobulin Levels	Associated Infections
GCs	Multiple antiinflammatory and autoimmune diseases	• Effect innate and acquired immunity via expression of multiple genes • Dose-dependent GS effects	• More significant effect on T cells compared with B cells • Hypogammaglobulinemia typically mild and not clinically significant • At high doses and chronic use: decrease number of peripheral B cells and decrease IgG and IgA levels • More significant hypogammaglobulinemia, caused by combination of glucocorticoids with other immunosuppressive medications	• Mild and severe bacterial, fungal, and viral infections • More common and more severe when GS are used with other immunosuppressive medications
Sulfasalazine	Rheumatoid arthritis, ulcerative colitis, other autoimmune diseases	• Exact mechanism of action unknown	• Inhibits neutrophil migration and reduces lymphocyte responses • Selective IgA deficiency • Reversible hypogammaglobulinemia, typically asymptomatic • Anemia, leukopenia	• Sepsis, pneumonia, no specific pathogens reported
Methotrexate	Acute lymphoid leukemia, juvenile idiopathic and rheumatoid arthritis, severe psoriasis	• Antimetabolite • Interferes with DNA synthesis, repair, and cellular replication by inhibiting dihydrofolate reductase	• Decreases immunoglobulin levels (rare) and antibody synthesis • Cytopenias • In high doses, causes profound bone marrow suppression	• Predominantly opportunistic infections, such as *Pneumocystis jiroveci* pneumonia, cryptococcosis, CMV disease (including pneumonia, sepsis), nocardiosis, herpes simplex and zoster infections, histoplasmosis • Bacterial infections, when used in combination with steroids

(continued on next page)

Table 1
(continued)

	Use	Mechanism of Action	Adverse Effects on Immune Cells and Immunoglobulin Levels	Associated Infections
Azathioprine (active form: 6-mercaptopurin)	Rheumatoid arthritis, systemic lupus erythematosus, other autoimmune diseases, transplant rejection	• Purine analogue of guanine and hypoxanthine	• Decreases T- and B-cell numbers, B-cell proliferation, antibody formation, and NK cell activity • Myelosuppression, predominantly leukopenia, hepatitis, and lymphoproliferative disorders	• Bacterial, viral, fungal, protozoal, opportunistic infections • Rate of infections significantly higher in patients who had renal transplants compared with those with rheumatoid arthritis
Mycophenolate mofetil (active form: mycophenolic acid)	Autoimmune hepatitis, refractory autoimmune cytopenias, lupus nephritis, myasthenia gravis, transplant rejection	• Blocks the production of guanine nucleotides required for DNA synthesis	• Inhibits T- and B-cell proliferation, recruitment of lymphocytes into areas of inflammation and antibody production by B lymphocytes • Leukopenia, other cytopenias, increased risk of lymphoproliferative disorders and skin cancers • Hypogammaglobulinemia, especially in combination with other immunomodulators	• Predominantly opportunistic infections, such as CMV, *Pneumocystis jiroveci*, nocardiosis, histoplasmosis, cryptococcosis, reactivation of polyoma viruses, herpes zoster and simplex viruses • Bacterial infections, especially with concomitant GCs
Cyclophosphamide, chlorambucil, melphalan	Different types of leukemia and lymphoma, multiple myeloma, cancers, autoimmune diseases, minimal change disease	• Alkylating agents • Cross-link strands of DNA and RNA and inhibit protein synthesis • Inhibition cholinesterase activity	• T- and B-cell lymphopenia • Suppressed antibody responses • Cytopenias, myelodysplastic syndrome • Secondary malignancies	• Bacterial, fungal (*Pneumocystis jiroveci*), viral (herpes zoster), protozoal, parasitic (*Strongyloides*) infections • Reactivation of latent infections

Abbreviations: CMV, cytomegalovirus; GCs, glucocorticoids; NK, natural killer.

BIOLOGICAL THERAPIES THAT CAUSE HYPOGAMMAGLOBULINEMIA

Biologics are large molecule therapeutics, usually proteins, which are isolated from human (or sometimes other biological) material or produced by in vitro cell culture or cell lines and recombinant gene technology. They include vaccines, blood and blood components, cellular therapies, gene therapy, tissues, and recombinant therapeutic proteins.[14] Immunosuppressive biological agents selectively target specific cytokines and/or block their receptors, typically with high affinity. The therapeutic precision of these drugs is very useful in the treatment of specific underlying diseases; but it can cause a profound deficiency of the targeted immunologic mediator, mimicking the disease observed in patients with PIDDs with homozygous genetic deletions of these mediators (**Table 2**).

Anti-CD20 Monoclonal Antibodies

Rituximab is a chimeric antibody against CD20 that selectively targets B cells and induces complete depletion of circulating and tissue-based CD201 B lymphocytes. It is widely used to treat malignant and autoimmune diseases. Early clinical trials demonstrated mild, transient hypogammaglobulinemia during the treatment with rituximab,[15] with an average B-cell recovery of 6 to 9 months after completion of therapy, with no significant increase in infection rate.[16,17] However, with expanding use of rituximab, its use in maintenance drug regimens, in combination with other immunosuppressive medications, and the availability of longer follow-up data, it has become clear that some patients treated with rituximab develop long-lasting B-cell immunosuppression. T-cell lymphopenia, predominantly affecting $CD4^+$ T cells has been reported as well.[18] It can be persistent and more prominent with maintenance regimens.[19] Depending on the study, up to 56% of rituximab-treated patients are reported to develop hypogammaglobulinemia with predominantly decreased IgG and immunoglobulin M (IgM) serum levels.[20,21] For the most part, hypogammaglobulinemia is mild, but some of these patients develop severe infections that require temporary or long-term immunoglobulin replacement therapy (IGRT).[22–24] Severe cytomegalovirus (CMV) infection, reactivation of latent hepatitis B infection and fatal progressive multifocal leukoencephalopathy were described with rituximab. In a study of 211 patients with non–Hodgkin lymphoma, 39% developed new onset decreased serum IgG and 72% of patients with preexisting low serum IgG had worsening of their hypogammaglobinemia. Seven percent developed symptomatic hypogammaglobinemia, defined by recurrent non-neutropenic infections.[25] Similar findings of post–rituximab hypogammaglobulinemia and increased severe infections were also reported in patients with rheumatoid arthritis,[22,26,27] multisystem autoimmune disease,[27] antineutrophil cytoplasmic antibody-associated vasculitis,[28] systemic lupus erythematosus,[29] and multiple myeloma[30] and in patients with neuroinflammatory diseases.[31]

Retrospective studies of patients with recurrent or severe infections and hypogammaglobulinemia requiring IGRT after rituximab treatment found persistent B-cell abnormalities.[32,33] Makatsori and colleagues[32] found that all 19 patients had reduced or absent B cells, reduced specific antibody levels, no response to *Haemophilus influenza B* (HIB), tetanus, and pneumococcal vaccinations, and needed IGRT for a mean of 36 months (range 7 months to 7 years) after the last rituximab dose. In the other study, 45% (5 of 11) of patients had persistently undetectable $CD19^+$ B cells (<3 cells) 9 to 31 months after receiving rituximab.[33] B-cell recovery in the rest of the patients was delayed with an average reconstitution time of 23 months after the last dose of rituximab. Furthermore, B-cell subpopulations after rituximab treatment were skewed toward naive B cells; there was a significant decrease in switched and memory B cells

Table 2
Biological agents that cause secondary hypogammaglobulinemia

Medication	Target	Selected Indications	Immunologic Effects	Infectious Complications
Rituximab	• Anti-CD20 chimeric monoclonal antibody	CLL NHL AAV RA	• B-cell depletion • Hypogammaglobulinemia • Decreased antibody responses to vaccinations	• Potentially fatal bacterial, fungal, and viral infections (CMV, herpes simplex, varicella zoster, parvovirus B19, West Nile, hepatitis B and C); PML due to JC virus infection • Reactivation of hepatitis B several months after completion of therapy
Ofatumumab	• Second-generation anti-CD20 human monoclonal antibody • Binds to a unique, more membrane proximal epitope of the CD20 and has been shown to be more potent than rituximab in preclinical models	Initial treatment as well as relapsed and refractory CLL	• B-cell depletion • Hypogammaglobulinemia (5%) in clinical trials	• 65%–70% incidence of bacterial, viral, and fungal infections, including sepsis (8%–10%) • Reactivation of hepatitis B several months after completion of therapy
Obinutuzumab	• Third-generation humanized anti-CD20 monoclonal antibody • More potent activity through antibody-dependent cellular cytotoxicity and direct B-cell apoptosis than rituximab	CLL, follicular lymphoma	• Limited data • B-cell depletion	• Limited data • Incidence of infection: 38%, including fatal and serious bacterial, fungal, and viral (herpes virus) infections

Drug	Mechanism	Indication	Effect	Infections
Alemtuzumab	• Recombinant monoclonal antibody specific for CD52 (Campath-1 antigen), which is present on many mature immune cells (T and B cells, NK cells, eosinophils, neutrophils, monocytes/macrophages, and dendritic cells) • Causes antibody-dependent cellular and complement-mediated lysis	Relapsing remitting multiple sclerosis, CLL, renal transplant rejection	• Reduction in B, T, NK cells and neutropenia early in treatment, persists for 4 to 9 mo after stopping therapy	• Bacterial, viral, fungal, and protozoal (*Listeria*) infections • CMV reactivation and infection • Reactivation of hepatitis B or hepatitis C, herpes, human papilloma virus, and tuberculosis • Also, increased risk of secondary autoimmune disease (30%–40%) and infections, including bacterial, fungal, *Listeria monocytogenes*
Belimumab	Anti-BLys humanized monoclonal antibody	SLE	• Alters B cells' survival and reduces the differentiation of B cells into immunoglobulin-producing plasma cells	Pneumonia, urinary tract infection, cellulitis, and bronchitis
Atacicept	Humanized fusion protein that binds Blys and APRIL	—	• Decreased numbers of mature and total circulating B cells and serum IgG, IgM, and IgA	Phase II/III trial in lupus nephritis stopped because of low immunoglobulin levels and pneumonias in some patients

Abbreviations: AAV, ANCA-associated vasculitis; BLys, B-lymphocyte stimulator; CLL, chronic lymphoid leukemia; CMV, cytomegalovirus; NHL, non-Hodgkin lymphoma; NK, natural killer; PML, progressive multifocal leukoencephalopathy; RA, rheumatoid arthritis; SLE, systemic lupus erythematosus.

in all of the patients. All patients had persistently low serum IgG levels with associated low IgA and IgM in 78% and 89% of these patients, respectively. None of these patients achieved an adequate response to *Streptococcus pneumoniae* polysaccharide vaccination (PPSV23). At 3.4 years after rituximab treatment (range, 1.0–6.5 years), 82% of patients were still requiring IGRT.[33]

Several factors associated with significant, symptomatic, persistent hypogammaglobinemia after rituximab have been described (see **Table 3**).[22–24,26–31,34–36] These include low baseline immunoglobulin levels, low CD19 count, more rituximab doses administered, use of other immunosuppressive drugs, older age, underlying disease treated with rituximab and concomitant medical conditions, or a combination of these risk factors.

The impact of rituximab on vaccination responses has been evaluated as well. Significantly decreased antibody responses were found to PPSV23, HIB,[37] and influenza A[38] vaccines within 6 months after CD20-depleting therapy. In patients with rheumatoid arthritis, antibody responses to influenza vaccination, administered 4 to 8 weeks after rituximab therapy, were significantly reduced compared with methotrexate-treated patients and healthy controls.[39] Humoral response improved, although it was still partial, when immunization was given 6 to 10 months after rituximab therapy, even in the absence of the repopulation of B cells. Another study of patients with rheumatoid arthritis measured vaccine responses after rituximab and methotrexate therapy for 36 weeks, compared with receiving methotrexate alone for 12 weeks. The investigators found similar tetanus toxoid responses in both groups but significantly decreased responses to PPSV23 and keyhole limpet hemocyanin (KLH, protein neoantigen) vaccines in the rituximab-treated group.[40] Antibody responses in 46 patients with newly diagnosed type 1 diabetes mellitus who completed 4 doses of rituximab and received no other IST showed protective, although significantly blunted, responses to tetanus, diphtheria. and hepatitis A immunizations 12 months after rituximab treatment compared with the placebo group.[41]

In an effort to further improve the therapeutic efficacy of rituximab, newer anti-CD20 monoclonal antibodies have been developed, such as ofatumumab, ocrelizumab, and obinutuzumab. Reactivation of hepatitis B has also been reported following anti-CD20 monoclonal antibody therapy. The Food and Drug Administration recommends screening all patients for hepatitis B virus (HBV) infection before starting treatment with ofatumumab and rituximab and monitoring patients who had prior HBV infection for clinical and laboratory signs of hepatitis B or HBV reactivation during and several months after treatment.[41]

Other Immunomodulatory Biologics

Other immunomodulatory biologics, such as monoclonal antibodies to cytokines that inhibit B-cell function (belimumab) and T-cell antigens (alemtuzumab),[42,43] are used in the setting of inflammatory disorders and have a potential of causing hypogammaglobulinemia (see **Table 2**). Abatacept downregulates T-cell activation by binding to CD80 and CD86 receptors on antigen-presenting cells and disrupts CD28 costimulation of T cells. It has not been associated with hypogammaglobulinemia; however, abatacept-treated patients with rheumatoid arthritis demonstrated significantly decreased serotype-specific IgG responses to PPSV23 compared with controls, while preserving opsonization responses, measured by multiplexed opsonophagocytic killing assay.[44] Belatacept is a second-generation CTLA-4-Ig fusion protein that has superior binding to CD80 and CD86 compared with abatacept, used in patients with renal transplants. Antithymocyte globulin

Table 3
Risk factors for postrituximab hypogammaglobulinemia and severe infections

Postrituximab Complications	Risk Factors	Underlying Disease	Notes	References
Hypogammaglobulinemia	• Low baseline IgG levels[a]	MAID	Weak association with cyclophosphamide exposure, but not cumulative rituximab dose	Roberts et al,[21] 2015
		RA	—	De La Torre et al,[27] 2012
			IgG levels <8 g/L	Boleto et al,[26] 2018
		Lymphoma	—	Filanovsky et al,[34] 2016
	• Low IgG levels at the time of rituximab	MAID	—	Roberts et al,[21] 2015
	• + Methotrexate	RA	—	Boleto et al,[26] 2018
	• Rituximab >8 doses	Lymphoma	—	Filanovsky et al,[34] 2016
	• + Fludarabine	Lymphoma	—	Filanovsky et al,[34] 2016
	• Prior purine exposure	Non-Hodgkin lymphoma	—	Casulo et al,[25] 2013
	• Heavily pretreated patients			
Low IgM	• Baseline serum IgM ≤0.8 g/L	Systemic lupus erythematosus	—	Reddy et al,[23] 2017
	• +Mycophenolate mofetil			

(continued on next page)

Table 3
(continued)

Postrituximab Complications	Risk Factors	Underlying Disease	Notes	References
Infections	• Lower IgG levels[a] • Lower CD19 counts • Creatinine clearance ≤45 mL/min[a] • Older age • Diabetes mellitus • Prednisone dosage >15 mg/d	Systemic autoimmune disease (RA excluded)	History of pneumococcal vaccination significantly *decreased* the risk of serious bacterial infections events	Heusele et al,[24] 2014
	• Baseline IgG level <6 g/L[a] • Chronic lung disease and/or cardiac insufficiency • Extra-articular involvement	RA	—	Gottenberg et al,[35] 2010
	• Low IgG	RA	Infection rates higher in low-IgG patients even before they developed low IgG	van Vollenhoven et al,[22] 2013
	• Reduction in IgM after rituximab • Duration of rituximab • G-CSF administration	Hematology patients	—	Kanbayashi et al,[36] 2009
	• IgG ≤375 • Low IgA	Granulomatosis with polyangiitis	IgG ≤375 associated with 23 times higher odds of infection, requiring hospitalization	Shah et al,[28] 2017
	• +Fludarabine • Female sex	Lymphoma	—	Cabanillas et al,[20] 2006
	• +Fludarabine • Secondary prolonged hypogammaglobulinemia	Lymphoma	—	Filanovsky et al,[34] 2016
	• Secondary hypogammaglobulinemia	RA	—	Boleto et al,[26] 2018

Abbreviations: G-CSF, granulocyte-colony stimulating factor; MAID, multisystem autoimmune disease; RA, rheumatoid arthritis.
[a] Baseline levels refer to levels before rituximab treatment.

(ATG) causes depletion of both T and B cells and is associated with increased herpes virus infections. There are no reports of ATG-induced hypogammaglobulinemia.

MALIGNANCIES AND HYPOGAMMAGLOBULINEMIA

While evaluating patients with suspected medication-induced hypogammaglobulinemia, it is important to remember that underlying illnesses like malignancies, particularly lymphoproliferative disorders, such as chronic lymphoid leukemia (CLL) and multiple myeloma (MM), are causes of SID. The incidence of hypogammaglobulinemia in CLL increases with disease duration and is present in up to 85% of patients at some point in their disease course, and severe infections are the major cause of death in 25% to 50% of patients with CLL.[45,46] Infection is also a major cause of morbidity and mortality in MM.[47] Malignancy-associated immunodeficiency with hypogammaglobulinemia is multifactorial. It involves various pathways of the immune system and is compounded by the treatment modalities used to manage these diseases. Splenectomy, immunosuppressive, antiinflammatory, and biological drugs, as well as underlying medical conditions/complications associated with malignancies, such as cytopenias, cardiac and pulmonary pathology, protein-losing nephropathy and gastroenteropathy, metabolic diseases, such as diabetes and uremia, all exponentially magnify SID in these patients. Identifying patients at risk for serious or recurrent infections secondary to hypogammaglobulinemia and treating them appropriately and prophylactically play a key role in preventing serious infections, which is a major cause of poor outcomes in patients with hematologic malignancies. Early vaccination, antiinfection prophylaxis, and replacement immunoglobulin are important preventative components.[48]

AFTER SOLID ORGAN TRANSPLANTATION

The risk of infection in organ transplant patients is governed by the "the net state of immunosuppression" and the epidemiologic exposures of the individual.[49] Many factors influence the "net state of immunosuppression," including type, dose, duration, and timeline of IST; host factors, such as underlying diseases and comorbidities, cytopenias, hypogammaglobulinemia and metabolic problems; the presence of devitalized tissues or fluid collections in the transplanted organ; and the presence of invasive devices and concomitant infection with immunomodulating viruses.[50–53] Transplant-associated IST increases the risk of nosocomial, community-acquired, and donor-derived infections and leads to reactivation and acceleration of latent, residual, and opportunistic infections. Hypogammaglobulinemia is one of numerous immunologic manifestations of transplant-associated immunosuppression. Hypogammaglobulinemia and low specific titers to PPSV23 and CMV were demonstrated to be risk factors for severe bacterial infections and CMV disease in heart transplant patients.[54] As rituximab is increasingly used for prevention and treatment of posttransplant lymphoproliferative disorders[55–57] and ABO blood group incompatibility,[58,59] the incidence of hypogammaglobulinemia is likely to increase. Identifying and addressing pretransplant and IST-related hypogammaglobulinemia along with widely used antimicrobial prophylaxis may decrease the rate of infections and improve outcomes.

EVALUATION AND MANAGEMENT OF HUMORAL DEFECT IN SECONDARY IMMUNODEFICIENCIES

Antibody deficiency is characterized not solely by abnormal immunoglobulin levels but also by the inability to mount primary and/or amnestic protective antibody responses to vaccinations and infectious antigens. Vaccines typically used by immunologists to identify antibody responses are tetanus toxoid and diphtheria toxin, HIB, and polysaccharide and conjugated pneumococcal (PCV13) vaccines as well as viral (measles, mumps, rubella, varicella) and neoantigen vaccines, such as φX174 and KLH. Although the administration of live viral vaccines is not appropriate in many immunodeficient patients, and neoantigen vaccines are not widely available, responses to tetanus toxoid, HIB, PPSV23, and PCV13 provide useful information in the management of patients with SID. B-cell phenotyping may be helpful in identifying patients with persistent humoral immune dysfunction caused by anti-CD20 therapies alone or compounded by preexistent immune defect of an underlying disease, such as PIDD, malignancy, and autoimmune disease.[32,60]

When evaluating patients with SID, it is also important to remember that autoimmune and some monoclonal proliferative diseases often are associated with hypergammaglobulinemia. The normal pretreatment and posttreatment immunoglobulin levels may be inadequately low for some of these patients, in line with the concept of the biological trough,[61] as characterized in PIDD. Additionally, patients treated with rituximab usually maintain protective specific antibody levels to the antigens they were exposed to before the treatment with a B-cell depleting drug, as immunoglobulin-producing plasma cells lose the CD20 cell surface marker during differentiation. However, these patients may not be able to mount appropriate responses to new infectious antigens or vaccines not received before B-cell depleting therapy and are at risk for infectious complications.

Management of SID includes screening for infections before starting immunomodulatory agents (for example, hepatitis B, CMV), early vaccinations, antiinfective prophylaxis, and replacement immunoglobulin when indicated. Reducing IST and treatment interruption in patients receiving immunosuppressive biologics should be considered if new infection develops. Patients with a history of recurrent and/or severe bacterial infections in the setting of hypogammaglobulinemia, poor responses to vaccinations, or failure to maintain vaccine titers should have a trial of IGRT to prevent further infections. Although optimal doses of IGRT in SID have not been established, the typical starting dosage is 350 to 400 mg/kg/mo (up to 600 mg/kg/mo in patients with bronchiectasis). The dose of intravenous or subcutaneous immunoglobulin should be adjusted to the lowest effective dose depending on the clinical response. The authors have adapted suggested protocols for the investigation, monitoring, and management of antibody failure in patients with CLL for use in patients with SID[62] (**Fig. 1**).

DISCUSSION AND FUTURE DIRECTIONS

SID, specifically hypogammaglobulinemia, is complex and multifactorial, involving multiple immune pathways. The use of immunomodulatory therapies and HSC or organ transplantation transformed the lives of countless patients, allowing the significant chance of a sustainable remission or total cure of a wide variety of diseases that, otherwise, had grave or fatal prognoses. As we accumulate knowledge and develop a clearer understanding of the immune mechanisms of the diseases themselves and the medical interventions that lead to SID, we must be continuously mindful that we should suspect, recognize, and treat early the underlying components of SID that can lead to serious, life-threatening, or fatal infections. It is important to remember that the immunosuppressive effects of medications may occur not only during or immediately after their use but can also manifest months or years after completion of this therapy. Drug-induced immunosuppression may be persistent and require long-term treatment with IGRT. Although not every patient with hypogammaglobulinemia will develop recurrent or serious infections, our role as clinicians is to identify patients at risk, as well as symptomatic patients with antibody deficiencies, and then institute appropriate, timely treatment.

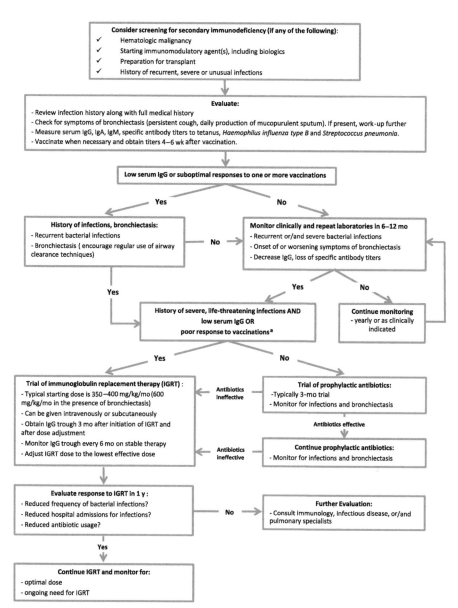

Fig. 1. Suggested protocol for work-up and management of humoral defect in SID. [a] It is a clinical decision whether or not to try antibiotic prophylaxis first or to go directly to IGRT. Patients treated with anti-CD20 agents may have protective preexisting-specific antibody titers but fail to generate new vaccine responses. (*Adapted from* Dhalla F, Lucas M, Schuh A, et al. Antibody deficiency secondary to chronic lymphocytic leukemia: should patients be treated with prophylactic replacement immunoglobulin? J Clin Immunol 2014;34(3):280; with permission.)

The natural history and management of SID vary depending on the causes of SID, thus, underscoring the need for further studies. For example, the characteristics and prognosis of SID secondary to lymphoma is different from that of chronic ITP treated with pulse steroids and rituximab. To differentiate between SID secondary to underlying illness and medication-induced immunodeficiency, the authors proposed the term *persistent immunodeficiency after treatment with immunomodulatory drugs*.[33] Obtaining baseline immunologic studies, such as serum IgG, IgA, IgM levels, selected specific antibody titers, and, when appropriate, immunophenotyping of peripheral blood lymphocytes in patients with hematologic malignancies, or before starting immunomodulatory agents and transplant therapy, is critical to identify a previously undiagnosed PIDD and help predict whether a given patient is at a higher risk of developing SID. It will allow clinicians to treat patients promptly, avoid recurrent and serious infectious complications, and help the development of an accurate prognosis. New controlled trials are needed to identify risk factors for patients who are likely to develop symptomatic SID and the efficacy, safety, and cost-effectiveness of the treatment of these patients with prophylactic antimicrobials and IGRT.

ACKNOWLEDGMENTS

The authors thank Galina Marder for critical reading of the article.

REFERENCES

1. Bonilla F. Practice parameter for the diagnosis and management of primary immunodeficiency. J Allergy Clin Immunol 2015;136(5):1186–205.
2. Chinen J, Shearer W. Secondary immunodeficiencies, including HIV infection. J Allergy Clin Immunol 2008;121(2S):S388–92.
3. Ashrafi M, Hosseini SA, Abolmaali S, et al. Effect of anti-epileptic drugs on serum immunoglobulin levels in children. Acta Neurol Belg 2010;110(1):65–70.
4. Abe S, Suzuki T, Hori T, et al. Hypogammaglobulinemia during antipsychotic therapy. Psychiatry Clin Neurosci 1998;52(1):115–7.
5. Svalheim S, Mushtaq U, Mochol M, et al. Reduced immunoglobulin levels in epilepsy patients treated with levetiracetam, lamotrigine, or carbamazepine. Acta Neurol Scand Suppl 2013;(196):11–5.
6. Maruyama S, Okamoto Y, Toyoshima M, et al. Immunoglobulin A deficiency following treatment with lamotrigine. Brain Dev 2016;38(10):947–9.
7. Smith J, Fernando T, McGrath N, et al. Lamotrigine-induced common variable immune deficiency. Neurology 2004;62(5):833–4.
8. Bousfiha AA, Jeddane L, Ailal F, et al. Primary immunodeficiency diseases worldwide: more common than generally thought. J Clin Immunol 2013;33(1):1–7.
9. Dixon WG, Abrahamowicz M, Beauchamp ME, et al. Immediate and delayed impact of oral glucocorticoid therapy on risk of serious infection in older patients with rheumatoid arthritis: a nested case-control analysis. Ann Rheum Dis 2012; 71(7):1128.
10. Berger W, Pollock J, Kiechel F, et al. Immunoglobulin levels in children with chronic severe asthma. Ann Allergy 1978;41(2):67–74.
11. Lack G, Ochs HD, Gelfand EW. Humoral immunity in steroid-dependent children with asthma and hypogammaglobulinemia. J Pediatr 1996;129(6):898.
12. Chen JY, Wang LK, Feng PH, et al. Risk of shingles in adults with primary Sjogren's syndrome and treatments: a nationwide population-based cohort study. PLoS One 2015;10(8):e0134930.
13. Yap DY, Yung S, Ma MK, et al. Serum immunoglobulin G level in patients with lupus nephritis and the effect of treatment with corticosteroids and mycophenolate mofetil. Lupus 2014;23(7):678–83.

14. What are "biologics" questions and answers. Available at: https://www.fda.gov/AboutFDA/CentersOffices/OfficeofMedicalProductsandTobacco/CBER/ucm133077.htm. Accessed April 21, 2018.
15. Maloney DG, Grillo-Lopez AJ, Bodkin DJ, et al. IDEC-C2B8: results of a phase I multiple-dose trial in patients with relapsed non-Hodgkin's lymphoma. J Clin Oncol 1997;15:3266–74.
16. David TA, White CA, Grillo-Lopez AJ, et al. Single-agent monoclonal antibody efficacy in bulky non-Hodgkin's lymphoma: results of a phase II trial of rituximab. J Clin Oncol 1999;17:1851–7.
17. Piro LT, White CA, Grillo-Lopez AJ, et al. Extended rituximab (anti CD20 monoclonal antibody) therapy for relapsed or refractory low-grade or follicular non-Hodgkin's lymphoma. Ann Oncol 1999;10:655–61.
18. Mélet J, Mulleman D, Goupille P, et al. Rituximab-induced T cell depletion in patients with rheumatoid arthritis: association with clinical response. Arthritis Rheum 2013;65(11):2783–90.
19. Yutaka T, Ito S, Ohigashi H, et al. Sustained CD4 and CD8 lymphopenia after rituximab maintenance therapy following bendamustine and rituximab combination therapy for lymphoma. Leuk Lymphoma 2015;56(11):3216–8.
20. Cabanillas F, Liboy I, Pavia O, et al. High incidence of non-neutropenic infections induced by rituximab plus fludarabine and associated with hypogammaglobulinemia: a frequently unrecognized and easily treatable complication. Ann Oncol 2006;17(9):1424–7.
21. Roberts DM, Jones RB, Smith RM, et al. Rituximab-associated hypogammaglobulinemia: incidence, predictors and outcomes in patients with multi-system autoimmune disease. J Autoimmun 2015;57:60–5.
22. van Vollenhoven RF, Emery P, Bingham CO, et al. Long term safety of rituximab in rheumatoid arthritis: 9.5-year follow-up of the global clinical trial programme with a focus on adverse events of interest in RA patients. Ann Rheum Dis 2013;72(9):1496–502.
23. Reddy V, Martinez L, Isenberg DA, et al. Pragmatic treatment of patients with systemic lupus erythematosus with rituximab: long-term effects on serum immunoglobulins. Arthritis Care Res (Hoboken) 2017;69(6):857–66.
24. Heusele M, Clerson P, Guery B, et al. Risk factors for severe bacterial infections in patients with systemic autoimmune diseases receiving rituximab. Clin Rheumatol 2014;33(6):799–805.
25. Casulo C, Maragulia J, Zelenetz AD. Incidence of hypogammaglobulinemia in patients receiving rituximab and the use of intravenous immunoglobulin for recurrent infections. Clin Lymphoma Myeloma Leuk 2013;13:106–11.
26. Boleto G, Avouac J, Wipff J, et al. Predictors of hypogammaglobulinemia during rituximab maintenance therapy in rheumatoid arthritis: a 12-year longitudinal multi-center study. Semin Arthritis Rheum 2018. https://doi.org/10.1016/j.semarthrit.2018.02.010.
27. De La Torre I, Leandro MJ, Valor L, et al. Total serum immunoglobulin levels in patients with RA after multiple B-cell depletion cycles based on rituximab: repletion with B-cell kinetics. Rheumatology 2012;51:833–40.
28. Shah S, Jaggi K, Greenberg K, et al. Immunoglobulin levels and infection risk with rituximab induction for anti-neutrophil cytoplasmic antibody-associated vasculitis. Clin Kidney J 2017;10(4):470–4.
29. Aguiar R, Araújo C, Martins-Coelho G, et al. Use of rituximab in systemic lupus erythematosus: a single center experience over 14 years. Arthritis Care Res 2017;69(2):257–62.

30. Vacca A, Melaccio A, Sportelli A, et al. Clin Immunol Subcutaneous immunoglobulins in patients with multiple myeloma and secondary hypogammaglobulinemia: a randomized trial. Clin Immunol 2018;191:110–5.

31. Tallantyre EC, Whittam DH, Jolles S, et al. Secondary antibody deficiency: a complication of anti-CD20 therapy for neuroinflammation. J Neurol 2018. https://doi.org/10.1007/s00415-018-8812-0.

32. Makatsori M, Kiani-Alikhan S, Manson AL, et al. Hypogammaglobulinaemia after rituximab treatment-incidence and outcomes. QJM 2014;107(10):821–8.

33. Kaplan B, Kopyltsova Y, Khokhar A, et al. Rituximab and immune deficiency: case series and review of the literature. J Allergy Clin Immunol Pract 2014;2(5): 594–600.

34. Filanovsky K, Miller EB, Sigler E, et al. Incidence of profound hypogammaglobulinemia and infection rate in lymphoma patients following the combination of chemotherapy and rituximab. Recent Pat Anticancer Drug Discov 2016;11(2): 228–35.

35. Gottenberg JE, Ravaud P, Bardin T, et al. Risk factors for severe infections in patients with rheumatoid arthritis treated with rituximab in the autoimmunity and rituximab registry. Arthritis Rheum 2010;62(9):2625–32.

36. Kanbayashi Y, Nomura K, Fujimoto Y, et al. Risk factors for infection in haematology patients treated with rituximab. Eur J Haematol 2009;82(1):26–30.

37. Nazi I, Kelton JG, Larché M, et al. The effect of rituximab on vaccine responses in patients with immune thrombocytopenia. Blood 2013;122:1946–53.

38. Yri OE, Torfoss D, Hungnes O, et al. Rituximab blocks protective serologic response to influenza A (H1N1) 2009 vaccination in lymphoma patients during or within 6 months after treatment. Blood 2011;118(26):6769–71.

39. van Assen S, Holvast A, Benne CA, et al. Humoral responses after influenza vaccination are severely reduced in patients with rheumatoid arthritis treated with rituximab. Arthritis Rheum 2010;62(1):75–81.

40. Bingham CO 3rd, Looney RJ, Deodhar A, et al. Immunization responses in rheumatoid arthritis patients treated with rituximab: results from a controlled clinical trial. Arthritis Rheum 2010;62(1):64–74.

41. FDA Drug Safety Communication: boxed warning and new recommendations to decrease risk of hepatitis B reactivation with the immune-suppressing and anti-cancer drugs Arzerra (ofatumumab) and Rituxan (rituximab). Available at: https://www.fda.gov/drugs/drugsafety/ucm366406.htm. Accessed April 28, 2018.

42. Ruck T, Bittner S, Wiendl H, et al. Alemtuzumab in multiple sclerosis: mechanism of action and beyond. Int J Mol Sci 2015;16(7):16414–39.

43. O'Brien SM, Keating MJ, Mocarski ES. Updated guidelines on the management of cytomegalovirus reactivation in patients with chronic lymphocytic leukemia treated with alemtuzumab. Clin Lymphoma Myeloma 2006;7(2):125.

44. Migita K, Akeda Y, Akazawa M, et al. Effect of abatacept on the immunogenicity of 23-valent pneumococcal polysaccharide vaccination (PPSV23) in rheumatoid arthritis patients. Arthritis Res Ther 2015;17:357.

45. Hamblin TJ. Chronic lymphocytic leukaemia. Baillieres Clin Haematol 1987;1: 449–91.

46. Hamblin AD, Hamblin TJ. The immunodeficiency of chronic lymphocytic leukaemia. Br Med Bull 2008;87:49–62.

47. Perri RT, Hebbel RP, Oken MM. Influence of treatment and response status on infection risk in multiple myeloma. Am J Med 1981;71(6):935–40.

48. Friman V, Winqvist O, Blimark C, et al. Secondary immunodeficiency in lympho-proliferative malignancies. Hematol Oncol 2016;34(3):121–32.
49. Fishman JA, Issa NC. Infection in organ transplantation: risk factors and evolving patterns of infection. Infect Dis Clin North Am 2010;24(2):273–83.
50. Collins LA, Samore MH, Roberts MS, et al. Risk factors for invasive fungal infections complicating orthotopic liver transplantation. J Infect Dis 1994;170:644.
51. Hadley S, Karchmer AW. Fungal infections in solid organ transplant recipients. Infect Dis Clin North Am 1995;9:1045.
52. van den Berg AP, Klompmaker IJ, Haagsma EB, et al. Evidence for an increased rate of bacterial infections in liver transplant patients with cytomegalovirus infection. Clin Transplant 1996;10:224.
53. Issa NC, Fishman JA. Infectious complications of antilymphocyte therapies in solid organ transplantation. Clin Infect Dis 2009;48:772.
54. Sarmiento E, Jaramillo M, Calahorra L, et al. Evaluation of humoral immunity profiles to identify heart recipients at risk for development of severe infections: a multicenter prospective study. J Heart Lung Transplant 2017;36(5):529–39.
55. Elstrom RL, Andreadis C, Aqui NA, et al. Treatment of PTLD with rituximab or chemotherapy. Am J Transplant 2006;6(3):569.
56. Choquet S, Leblond V, Herbrecht R, et al. Efficacy and safety of rituximab in B-cell post-transplantation lymphoproliferative disorders: results of a prospective multicenter phase 2 study. Blood 2006;107(8):3053.
57. Trappe R, Oertel S, Leblond V, et al. Sequential treatment with rituximab followed by CHOP chemotherapy in adult B-cell post-transplant lymphoproliferative disorder (PTLD): the prospective international multicentre phase 2 PTLD-1 trial. Lancet Oncol 2012;13(2):196–206.
58. Vo AA, Choi J, Cisneros K, et al. Benefits of rituximab combined with intravenous immunoglobulin for desensitization in kidney transplant recipients. Transplantation 2014;98(3):312–9.
59. Lee EC, Kim SH, Shim JR, et al. A comparison of desensitization methods: rituximab with/without plasmapheresis in ABO-incompatible living donor liver transplantation. Hepatobiliary Pancreat Dis Int 2018;17(2):119–25.
60. Anolik JH, Friedberg JW, Zheng B, et al. B-cell reconstitution after rituximab treatment of lymphoma recapitulates B-cell ontogeny. Clin Immunol 2007;122:139–45.
61. Bonagura VR. Dose and outcomes in primary immunodeficiency disorders. Clin Exp Immunol 2014;178(S1):7–9.
62. Dhalla F, Lucas M, Schuh A, et al. Antibody deficiency secondary to chronic lymphocytic leukemia: should patients be treated with prophylactic replacement immunoglobulin? J Clin Immunol 2014;34:277–82.

An Update on Syndromes with a Hyper-IgE Phenotype

Jenna R.E. Bergerson, MD, MPH[a], Alexandra F. Freeman, MD[b],*

KEYWORDS

- Autosomal dominant hyper-IgE syndrome • Job's syndrome
- Signal transducer and activator of transcription 3
- Autosomal recessive hyper-IgE syndrome • Dedicator of cytokinesis 8
- ERBB2-interacting protein • Phosphoglucomutase 3

KEY POINTS

- Many primary immunodeficiencies disorders are associated with an elevated immunoglobulin E (IgE) level. With improvement in next-generation sequencing several new genetic causes have been found, expanding the number of syndromes associated with high IgE.
- Although there is clinical and immunologic overlap, there are important immunologic and nonimmunologic sequelae that help distinguish them.
- Infection control and prophylaxis are essential in these diseases, but some such as dedicator of cytokinesis 8 deficiency clearly justify hematopoietic stem cell transplantation.

INTRODUCTION

Hyperimmunoglobulin E (IgE) infection syndrome (HIES), also called Job's syndrome, was described in the 1970s in individuals with eczema, recurrent infections, and elevated serum IgE. Since that time, multiple distinct diseases, with the triad of eczema, infections, and high IgE, have been delineated with both autosomal dominant and recessive inheritance. Dominant negative mutations in signal transducer and activator of transcription 3 (*STAT3*) were identified in 2007 as the link between recurrent infections and connective tissue abnormalities in autosomal dominant HIES

Disclosures: The authors have no commercial or financial conflicts of interest to disclose.
This work was supported by the Intramural Research Program, National Institutes of Health Clinical Center. The content of this article does not necessarily reflect the views or policies of the Department of Health and Human Services, nor does mention of trade names, commercial products, or organizations imply endorsement by the US government.
[a] Laboratory of Clinical Immunology and Microbiology, National Institutes of Allergy and Infectious Diseases (NIAID), National Institutes of Health (NIH), 10 Center Drive, Building 10, Room 11N244a, Bethesda, MD 20892, USA; [b] Laboratory of Clinical Immunology and Microbiology, National Institutes of Allergy and Infectious Diseases (NIAID), National Institutes of Health (NIH), 10 Center Drive, Building 10, Room 12C103, Bethesda, MD 20892, USA
* Corresponding author.
E-mail address: freemaal@mail.nih.gov

Immunol Allergy Clin N Am 39 (2019) 49–61
https://doi.org/10.1016/j.iac.2018.08.007
0889-8561/19/© 2018 Elsevier Inc. All rights reserved.

immunology.theclinics.com

(AD-HIES).[1,2] More recently, two dominantly inherited disorders have been described; an *ERBB2IP* mutation, which encodes for the protein ERBIN, and CARD11 mutations.[3,4] Newly described autosomal recessive diseases include those due to mutations in phosphoglucomutase 3 (*PGM3*), dedicator of cytokinesis 8 (*DOCK8*), and interleukin 6 signal transducer (*IL6ST*).[5-8]

The different molecular and clinical manifestations of these distinct diseases with a hyper-IgE phenotype are reviewed here with a particular emphasis on loss-of-function (LOF) STAT3 mutations and DOCK8 deficiency.

AUTOSOMAL DOMINANT DISORDERS
Loss of Function STAT3

AD-HIES, Job's syndrome, is a primary immunodeficiency disorders caused by dominant-negative mutations in STAT3[1,2] and characterized by elevated IgE; eczema; infections; and multiple connective tissue, skeletal, and vascular abnormalities.

Immunologic and infectious complications

Pustular or eczematoid eruptions on the face and scalp typically begin in the first few weeks of life and persist frequently through the teenage years (**Fig. 1**). Exacerbations of the rash are often due to *Staphylococcus aureus*, and control of eczema is typically most successful with topical or systemic antistaphylococcal therapy. Characteristic "cold" abscesses usually start in early childhood but are minimized with *S aureus* control.

Recurrent pulmonary infections also manifest in early childhood and are predominantly due to infection with *S aureus*, *Streptococcus pneumoniae*, and *Haemophilus* species. Patients lack systemic inflammatory signs, which may delay diagnosis, but local airway inflammation and copious airway secretions are seen. Aberrant healing following lung infection frequently leads to bronchiectasis and pneumatoceles. Pulmonary nontuberculous mycobacteria infection occurs at a rate similar to that seen in cystic fibrosis, as does infection with gram-negative organisms such as *Pseudomonas aeruginosa* and filamentous molds such as Aspergillus and Scedosporium (**Fig. 2**A). These chronic infections are the cause of significant morbidity and mortality because antimicrobial resistance becomes problematic and hemoptysis risk increases.[9] Lung surgery, like pneumatocele resection, is frequently complicated by poor healing and bronchopleural fistulae.[10]

Although most of the pulmonary mold infections are seen in areas of preexisting parenchymal damage, occasionally features of allergic bronchopulmonary aspergillosis are seen. Making this diagnosis in a syndrome defined by high IgE levels is complicated due to falsely positive antigen-specific serologies, so the diagnosis

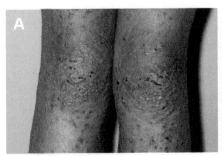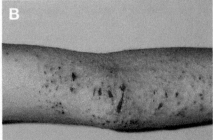

Fig. 1. (*A, B*) Chronic severe eczematous dermatitis in a 10-year-old with LOF STAT3.

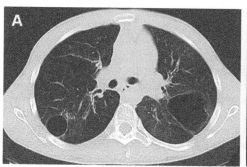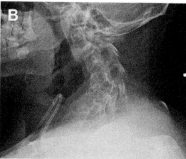

Fig. 2. Imaging findings in LOF STAT3 patients. (*A*) Pneumatoceles and bronchiectasis in a 29-year-old man. (*B*) Severe cervical spine kyphosis in a 37-year-old man.

must be made using typical radiographic findings in conjunction with clinical response to corticosteroids, antifungal therapy, and omalizumab treatment.

Mucocutaneous candidiasis can present as disease of the nails, oropharynx, esophagus, and vaginal mucosa. Opportunistic infections can also be seen in LOF STAT3; *Pneumocystis jiroveci* pneumonia (PJP) has been reported in infants presenting with their first pneumonia.[11] Endemic fungi can disseminate and lead to gastrointestinal (GI) disease, such as with Histoplasmosis and Cryptococcus, or meningitis, with Coccidiodes and Cryptococcus.[12]

Reactivation of viral infections, specifically varicella zoster virus (VZV), has been observed in this population at significantly increased rates. Nearly one-third of LOF STAT3 patients had a history of herpes zoster, starting at young ages. This impaired control of chronic viral infections is proposed to be due to the observed defect in central memory T cells seen in LOF STAT3 patients.[13]

Despite the elevated total and antigen-specific IgE, LOF STAT3 has less clinical food allergy and anaphylaxis compared with other highly atopic patients. The may be due to the role of STAT3 signaling, essential for mast cell mediator–induced vascular permeability, which is impaired in patients with LOF STAT3.[14]

An increased incidence of both Hodgkin and non-Hodgkin lymphoma is seen.[15,16] Despite issues with viral reactivation, there does not seem to be any relationship with Epstein–Barr virus (EBV) infection and malignancy in this population. Furthermore, as STAT3 is an oncogene, the development of lymphoma is paradoxical and further investigation is necessary to understand the mechanism of tumorigenesis within this population.

Nonimmunologic manifestations

Characteristic facial features usually manifest during adolescence and are characterized by a prominent forehead and chin, deep-set eyes, a broad nose, and porous skin.[17] A high-arched palate and failure to shed primary teeth is common.[18,19] An increased frequency of aphthous stomatitis is also seen during the teenage/early adolescent years (Alexandra Freeman, MD, unpublished observations).

Other musculoskeletal abnormalities include hyperextensible joints, scoliosis, minor trauma fractures, and osteopenia (**Fig. 2B**). Scoliosis is present in many patients and may be severe enough to warrant surgical correction. Unlike poor wound healing seen following pulmonary surgery, orthopedic surgeries are typically uncomplicated. Joints are typically hyperextensible, which perhaps explains the significant arthritis seen at younger ages than in the general population. Degenerative cervical spine disease in the fourth and fifth decade of life can cause neurologic deficits and may require surgical stabilization.

Vascular abnormalities include aneurysms, dilation and tortuosity of middle sized arteries such as coronary and cerebral arteries.[20] These can be symptomatic leading to myocardial infarction, subarachnoid hemorrhage, and intestinal hemorrhage. Our center routinely screens for coronary artery and cerebral aneurysm by magnetic resonance angiogram, starting in the late childhood and early adolescent years, repeating every three years. Coronary vessel walls were found to be significantly thicker in AD-HIES patient than in healthy subjects, which indicate atherosclerosis being present but not leading to narrowing, perhaps due to disordered tissue remodeling associated with STAT3 mutations.[21]

Central nervous system abnormalities are a more common finding on imaging as well.[22] Asymptomatic, focal white matter hyperintensities are seen on brain MRI in most individuals with LOF STAT3 and have an appearance similar to small vessel disease.[22,23] Chiari malformation type 1 and craniosynostosis have also been found in a higher incidence in AD-HIES patients, but generally have not required surgical correction.[22]

The GI manifestations in LOF STAT3 reflect both the immune abnormalities and the connective tissue findings. This includes infections of the GI tract with Candida and other endemic fungal organisms related to the impaired epithelial host immunity presumably. In one large cohort of patients, 60% of the patients reported one or more GI symptoms, with gastroesophageal reflux disease (GERD) and dysphagia being the most common. Chronic eosinophilic esophagitis (EoE) and underlying GI dysmotility may lead to food impaction. Colonic perforation in several patients likely related to abnormal mucosal and connective tissue repair. No increased incidence of inflammatory bowel disease (IBD) was seen, perhaps due to the absence of Th17 cells in STAT3-deficient patients, as increased IL-17 signaling has been observed in IBD.[24,25]

Laboratory Findings/Diagnostic Testing

The most consistent laboratory finding is an elevated serum IgE level. The peak is typically greater than 2000 IU/mL, but the level tends to decrease, or even normalize with increased age, and does not correlate with disease severity. The complete blood count is typically normal, but there can be relative neutropenia. The white blood cell count often fails to increase in response to infection and eosinophilia is also common. Although serum IgG and IgM are usually normal, and serum IgA is normal or low, specific antibody responses to encapsulated organisms can be impaired. Lymphocyte phenotyping often reveals diminished memory T and B cells and very low IL-17 producing T cells.

Pathophysiology

STAT3 has been shown to be essential for embryogenesis, as homozygous STAT3 knockout mice do not survive.[26] Most of the disease-causing mutations occur in the SH2 or the DNA-binding domains and are either short in-frame deletions or missense mutations that result in normal STAT3 protein expression but decreased function. Although there are no clear genotype-phenotype correlations, there is a modest increase in some of the nonimmunologic features, such as high palate, wide nose, and scoliosis in those with SH2 domain mutations.[27]

STAT3 is expressed widely and mediates various pathways involved in wound healing, host defense, and vascular remodeling, consistent with its multisystem clinical phenotype. Multiple cytokines transduce signal using STAT3, including IL-6, IL-10,

IL-11, IL-17, IL-21, IL-22, IL-23, leukemia inhibitory factor, oncostatin M, cardiotrophin-1, cardiotrophin-like cytokine, and ciliary neurotrophic factor. One of the defining immunologic abnormalities in this disease is failure of Th17 cells to differentiate, leading to impaired upregulation of antimicrobial peptides at epithelial surfaces, which results in Candida and S aureus infections.[25] Impaired IL-11 signaling has been shown to cause craniosynostosis, delayed tooth eruption, and supernumerary teeth in 3 consanguineous families in Pakistan with IL-11R alpha mutations due to lack of STAT3 transduction.[28]

STAT3 also plays an important role in the regulation of matrix metalloproteinases (MMPs), and as expected those with STAT3 deficiency have abnormal levels of MMP.[29] Such a defect in tissue remodeling likely explains the vascular aneurysms, poor lung healing after infection, and characteristic facial features with porous skin seen in this population.

Treatments/Prognosis

The main target of therapy for LOF STAT3 involves the prevention and treatment of infections. Earlier diagnosis of LOF STAT3 through greater recognition of clinical phenotype and genetic testing enable implementation of preventative antimicrobial therapies before development of significant comorbidities and are significantly improving the quality of life and life span of those affected. Because LOF STAT3 patients can lack the classic signs of infection, a careful history, physical examination, and relevant imaging are important to initiate timely therapies.

Prophylactic antibiotics targeting S aureus (eg, trimethoprim/sulfamethoxazole) are useful to decrease the frequency of pyogenic pneumonia, with the goal of preventing parenchymal lung disease. Control of skin disease, exacerbated by S aureus, also is benefited by oral antistaphylococcal therapy, along with topical antiseptics such as dilute bleach baths or chlorhexidine washes. Infections of the axilla and groin can persist, however, despite even aggressive skin care and decolonization of bacteria on the skin.

Antifungal prophylaxis may be of help in LOF STAT3 patients with chronic or recurrent Candida infections such as onychomycosis. Those who have evidence of mold colonization or infection of the lung should be treated with antifungal agents with activity against molds, such as posaconazole. Anti-Aspergillus prophylaxis should also be considered for any AD-HIES patient with pneumatoceles, because they are at higher risk for the development of aspergillomas. In areas with endemic mycoses, antifungal prophylaxis for Coccidioides and Histoplasma should be strongly considered.

Airway clearance techniques should be used as in other patients with bronchiectasis. However, the benefits that aggressive airway management can offer must be balanced by the increased risk of hemoptysis that some of these patients face, and in these cases oral antimicrobial therapy should be optimized and inhaled airway irritants should be withheld during acute episodes of hemoptysis. Also complicating the manner in which airway clearance is delivered is the increased risk for minimal trauma fractures, thus limiting the use of devices such as the percussive vest.[9]

Immunoglobulin replacement, administered by either intravenous or subcutaneous routes, can decrease the incidence of sinopulmonary infections and should be strongly considered in patients with recurrent pulmonary infections despite prophylactic antibiotics, parenchymal lung damage, or poor specific antibody production.[30]

Routine vaccination according to an age appropriate schedule is recommended. These vaccines are usually tolerated well, with the exception of the 23-valent pneumococcal vaccine in which a subset of individuals with LOF STAT3 have developed fever, and large areas of edema and erythema develop around the injection site, often times requiring systemic steroids (Alexandra Freeman, MD, unpublished observations). The pneumococcal conjugate vaccine has been well tolerated, but avoiding the 23-valent pneumococcal vaccine should be considered in this population.

Optimal therapy for GI disorders remains to be determined. Experience with the use of oral or topical corticosteroid therapy for EoE is limited in this population, and it is reasonable to be concerned about using such a therapy in these patients who are already prone to both infections and osteoporosis. The use of long-term acid suppression for GERD, with either proton pump inhibitors or H2 blockers, raises similar concerns.

The role of hematopoietic stem cell transplantation (HSCT) in LOF STAT3 is not straight forward because some of the disease manifestations are of nonhematopoietic origin. The first two reports of HSCT in AD-HIES patient were deemed failures due to complications in the posttransplant period.[31,32] Encouragingly, more recent reports of transplantation in this patient population indicate that HSCT may be an important therapeutic option in patients with severe disease manifestations. In some cases, improvement in immunologic and nonimmunologic features of the underlying disease has been reported.[33]

ERBIN deficiency

In 2017, Lyons and colleagues reported a family with an LOF mutation in *ERBB2IP*, which encodes for the protein ERBIN. Significant allergic and connective tissue features overlap with LOF STAT3, including elevated IgE, eosinophilic esophagitis, joint hypermobility, and vascular abnormalities. However, this family with ERBIN deficiency does not seem to have the mucosal susceptibility to candida, impairment in T- and B-cell memory, and defect in class-switching as is seen in LOF STAT3 patients.[3] The significant clinical overlap between patients with LOF STAT3 and these patients with ERBIN deficiency suggests a mechanistic link between these two proteins. STAT3 activation promotes ERBIN expression and negatively regulates transforming growth factor beta (TGF-β) activity by the formation of a STAT3/ERBIN/SMAD2/3 complex. In these ERBIN-deficient patients increased activation of the TGF-β pathway results in elevated numbers of T regulatory cells and functional IL4Rα expression on naïve lymphocytes. TGF-β can drive IL4/IL4R/GATA3 expression in vitro, and TGF-β–induced SMAD2/3 activity correlates with increased Th2 cytokine expressing memory cells and high IgE levels in LOF STAT3 and ERBIN-deficient patients.

LOF *CARD11* MUTATIONS

CARD11 (also known as *CARMA1*) encodes a membrane-associated guanylate kinase (MAGUK)-family protein, which partners with BCL10 and MALT1 to form a complex that is required for inhibitor of κβ kinase (IKK) and natural killer (NK)-κβ activation on lymphocyte receptor engagement. A spectrum of disease has been described for mutations in CARD11; homozygous null mutations in *CARD11* cause a form of severe combined immunodeficiency (SCID),[34] and heterozygous gain-of-function mutations result in a B-cell lymphoproliferative disease known as BENTA.[35]

Eight patients from four families with severe atopic dermatitis were identified with heterozygous hypomorphic *CARD11* mutations. The nonimmunologic manifestations seen in *STAT3, DOCK8, and PGM3* deficiencies are less prominent in these patients, but the severe atopic dermatitis, eosinophilia, and elevated IgE level are shared. Recurrent pulmonary infections were seen in most patients at a young age. Other atopic manifestations such as asthma, food allergy, and eosinophilic

GI disease were reported as well. In addition to the more prominent laboratory findings of high IgE and eosinophilia, B-cell lymphopenia, notably low-memory B cells, with decreased IgM, normal IgG, and normal to high IgA was reported. It has been proposed that the largely atopic phenotype observed in these patients is due to disruption of T-cell receptor, which has been associated with a Th2 bias. The attenuation of CARD11-dependent mTORC1 activation likely contributes to altered Th1 differentiation in these patients, allowing mTORC2-dependent Th2 responses to predominate.[4]

AUTOSOMAL RECESSIVE DISORDERS
DOCK8 Deficiency

DOCK8 deficiency is an autosomal recessive combined immunodeficiency syndrome associated with elevated IgE, recurrent sinopulmonary and cutaneous viral infections, atopy, and malignancies. In 2004, Renner and colleagues[36] reported patients with an autosomal recessive variant of HIES, but a genetic cause involving biallelic mutations often with large deletions was not described until 2009.[6,7]

Clinical presentation
Patients typically present with signs of atopic dermatitis, S aureus skin infections, pneumonias, elevated IgE, and eosinophilia. Typically, there are more allergic manifestations in DOCK8 deficiency than in LOF STAT3, including atopic dermatitis, food allergies, asthma, and eosinophilic esophagitis.

Unlike in LOF STAT3, there is susceptibility to cutaneous viral infections such as human papillomavirus (HPV) leading to widespread and recalcitrant warts, disseminated molluscum contagiosum, herpes simplex virus, and VZV (**Fig. 3**). Less commonly, other severe systemic viral infections have been seen such as cytomegalovirus disease or progressive multifocal leukoencephalopathy.[6,37,38]

Most patients also have a history of recurrent sinopulmonary infections, including PJP, and complications such as bronchiectasis formation occur in more than one-third of patients. Biliary tract–related liver disease due to cryptosporidium infection can be quite significant. However, significant liver disease not associated with cryptosporidium has also been reported.[39,40]

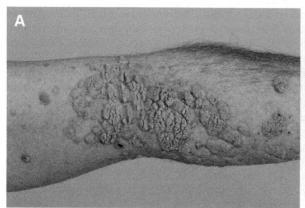
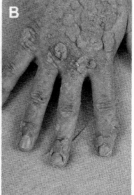

Fig. 3. (A, B) Large, widespread warts due to severe HPV infection in a 27-year-old man with DOCK8 deficiency.

Malignancy is a key feature of DOCK 8 deficiency and tends to be particularly aggressive and arises at a younger age.[37] Malignancies tend to be secondary to poor control of viruses such as HPV-associated squamous cell carcinomas and EBV-related lymphomas and smooth muscle tumors.[41] Cancers not typically associated with viral infections, such as microcystic adnexal carcinoma and rapidly progressive T-cell lymphoma, have also been found.[6]

Vascular abnormalities are thought to occur from vasculitis. Cerebral aneurysms and stenosis are seen and have been associated with stroke and moyamoya. Aortic and abdominal arterial vasculitis has been described. Other autoimmune conditions such as autoimmune hemolytic anemia occur rarely.[37,38]

Laboratory features

DOCK8 deficiency is a combined immunodeficiency involving both T and B cells, frequently with progressive lymphopenia over time. Memory B cells and switched memory B cells are almost completely absent in most DOCK8-deficient patients.[38,42] Naïve T cells and recent thymic emigrant T cells have been reported by one group to be low, with Th2 skewing seen as well.[42] Memory T cell numbers are variable, but in one study most CD8+ cells had an exhausted phenotype (CD45RA+/CCR7−).[38,43] Elevated IgE and eosinophilia are found in almost all of the patients. IgG tends to be either normal or elevated, IgA levels normal, and IgM levels are typically decreased and continued to decline with age. Vaccine responses to protein and polysaccharide antigens are variable.[37,41]

Pathophysiology

DOCK8 belongs to the DOCK180 superfamily of atypical guanine exchange factors involved in actin cytoskeleton regulation via activation of members of the Ras homolog gene family of small guanine triphosphate-binding proteins, such as Rac and Cdc42.

The importance of DOCK8 in controlling both actin cytoskeleton–dependent and independent immune responses is reflected in both innate and adaptive immunities. In a DOCK8 knockout murine model, dendritic cells (DCs) were unable to migrate through 3-dimensional space from the skin to local lymph nodes for T-cell priming due to impaired Cdc42 activation at the leading-edge membrane. Furthermore, deficiency of plasmacytoid DCs with poor interferon alpha (INF-α) levels is seen in the peripheral blood of DOCK8-deficient patients.[44,45]

The inability of the actin cytoskeleton to coordinate the accumulation of adhesion molecules and cytotoxic granules at immunologic synapses also contributes to impaired lymphocyte survival, NK cell–mediated cell killing, and memory responses. In addition, DOCK8 is necessary to control the actin cytoskeleton network as T and NK cells migrate through collagen-dense tissues such as skin. When this cannot occur, as in DOCK8 deficiency, a form of cell death occurs, called cytothripsis. The early cell death of T and NK cells prevents the generation of skin-resident memory CD8+ T cells and may explain the severe cutaneous viral infections seen in these patients.[43,46–48]

B cells from DOCK8-deficient mice lack marginal zone B cells, have difficulty surviving in germinal centers, and cannot undergo affinity maturation, resulting in poor persistence of antibody response following immunization. DOCK8 seems to be essential for recruitment of the integrin ligand ICAM-1, which is necessary for B-cell immunologic synapse formation.[49] DOCK8 additionally affects B-cell responses as an adaptor linking TLR9 to MyD88 and downstream signaling pathways to affect B-cell activation.[50] Recent work has shown that DOCK8 regulates B-cell receptor clustering, B-cell spreading, and activation of memory B cells by regulating CD19 and WAS protein expression.[51]

Treatment

DOCK8 deficiency is associated with significant morbidity and mortality with about half of patients dying before the age of 20 years. HSCT has been shown to be the only curative option for DOCK8 deficiency and is recommended at early stages of the disease. While awaiting definitive treatment with transplant, significant complications related to infection and malignancy must be aggressively managed. Antibacterial and antiviral prophylaxis is recommended, and immunoglobulin replacement therapy should also be strongly considered. Systemic INF-α 2b therapy, which may inhibit viral replication and activate effector lymphocytes, has shown efficacy in treating severe viral infections.[44,45] However, side effects can be significant and careful monitoring while on therapy is essential. Avoidance of potentially Cryptosporidium-contaminated water is prudent. Vascular imaging of cerebral vessels to detect areas of stenosis is essential to prevent stroke.

PGM3 Deficiency

In 2014, autosomal recessive hypomorphic mutations in PGM3 were described in nine kindreds by 3 independent groups. The clinical phenotype of the patients is quite variable and ranges from SCID to a hyper-IgE phenotype.[5,52,53] Hypomorphic PGM3 in mice results in a bone marrow failure phenotype, similar to the clinical phenotype observed in patients with deleterious PGM3 mutations who present early in life with a T-B-NK + SCID phenotype and neutropenia.[53–55] Other patients have more of an indolent course, with frequent sinopulmonary infections complicated by bronchiectasis, increased IgE levels, atopy, neurocognitive impairment, and autoimmunity (**Fig. 4**).[5,52] Connective tissue and skeletal abnormalities such as joint hyperextensibility, scoliosis, and short limbs have been reported. Unique to patients with PGM3 mutations and a hyper-IgE phenotype is an increase in Th17 cells and autoimmunity.[56]

To date, no clear treatment strategy has been identified and the efficacy of HSCT needs to be more fully evaluated. Many of the reported PGM3-deficient patients either succumbed to infection before HSCT or had such severe end-organ damage that HSCT was not a viable therapeutic option. However, two patients with an SCID-like phenotype were reported to successfully undergo HSCT with resolution of their lymphopenia and neutropenia.[53]

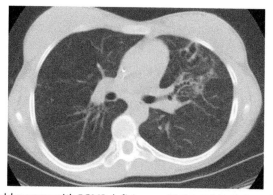

Fig. 4. A 21-year-old woman with PGM3 deficiency with bronchiectasis and scarring on chest computer tomography scan.

Pathophysiology

PGM3 deficiency is a congenital disorder of glycosylation (CDG). The widespread clinical manifestations are thought to be due to the pervasive role of glycosylation in normal cellular functions. CDGs have been described to cause immune defects because glycosylation is necessary for normal functioning of most immune receptors, immunoglobulins, complement proteins, and cytokines (reviewed in Ref.[56]). The phosphoglucomutases (PGMs) belong to a family of phosphohexose mutases that facilitate the conversion of glucose-1 phosphate to glucose-6-phosphate. The globally expressed human phosphoglucomutase 3 (PGM3) catalyzes a key step in the synthesis of uridine diphosphate N-acetylglucosamine, which is an essential precursor for protein glycosylation and critical to multiple glycosylation pathways.[5,52] Further work is underway to better understand how defects in these pathways cause such a profound effect on the immune system in particular.

IL6ST

More recently a patient with homozygous *IL6ST* mutations was described with manifestations including eczema, elevated IgE, and eosinophilia. Like *STAT3, DOCK8,* and *PGM3* mutations, this patient also presented with nonimmunologic manifestations of craniosynostosis and scoliosis. In addition, recurrent infections, bronchiectasis, decreased memory B cells, and an impaired acute-phase response were also described.

IL6ST encodes the evolutionarily conserved GP130 cytokine receptor subunit, which is necessary for signaling via IL-6, IL-11, IL-27, oncostatin M, and leukemia inhibitory factor. GP130-associated signaling is mediated by the JAK/STAT pathway and includes phosphorylation of STAT3 and STAT1, so with loss of GP130 there is not surprisingly significant overlap with LOF *STAT3* mutations.[8]

SUMMARY

Improvement in genetic testing has led to more specific diagnosis and delineation of immune dysregulation syndromes characterized by the hyper IgE phenotype of eczema, recurrent infections, and elevated serum IgE. Genetic testing is essential to predict the clinical course and determine the indication for therapies such as HSCT.

REFERENCES

1. Holland SM, DeLeo FR, Elloumi HZ, et al. STAT3 mutations in the hyper-IgE syndrome. N Engl J Med 2007;357(16):1608–19.
2. Minegishi Y, Saito M, Tsuchiya S, et al. Dominant-negative mutations in the DNA-binding domain of STAT3 cause hyper-IgE syndrome. Nature 2007;448(7157): 1058–62.
3. Lyons JJ, Liu Y, Ma CA, et al. ERBIN deficiency links STAT3 and TGF-beta pathway defects with atopy in humans. J Exp Med 2017;214(3):669–80.
4. Ma CA, Stinson JR, Zhang Y, et al. Germline hypomorphic CARD11 mutations in severe atopic disease. Nat Genet 2017;49(8):1192–201.
5. Zhang Y, Yu X, Ichikawa M, et al. Autosomal recessive phosphoglucomutase 3 (PGM3) mutations link glycosylation defects to atopy, immune deficiency, autoimmunity, and neurocognitive impairment. J Allergy Clin Immunol 2014;133(5): 1400–9, 1409.e1-5.
6. Zhang Q, Davis JC, Lamborn IT, et al. Combined immunodeficiency associated with *DOCK8* mutations. N Engl J Med 2009;361(21):2046–55.

7. Engelhardt KR, McGhee S, Winkler S, et al. Large deletions and point mutations involving the dedicator of cytokinesis 8 (DOCK8) in the autosomal-recessive form of hyper-IgE syndrome. J Allergy Clin Immunol 2009;124(6):1289–302.e4.
8. Schwerd T, Twigg SRF, Aschenbrenner D, et al. A biallelic mutation in IL6ST encoding the GP130 co-receptor causes immunodeficiency and craniosynostosis. J Exp Med 2017;214(9):2547–62.
9. Freeman AF, Olivier KN. Hyper-IgE syndromes and the lung. Clin Chest Med 2016;37(3):557–67.
10. Freeman AF, Renner ED, Henderson C, et al. Lung parenchyma surgery in autosomal dominant hyper-IgE syndrome. J Clin Immunol 2013;33(5):896–902.
11. Freeman AF, Davis J, Anderson VL, et al. Pneumocystis jiroveci infection in patients with hyper-immunoglobulin E syndrome. Pediatrics 2006;118(4):e1271–5.
12. Odio CD, Milligan KL, McGowan K, et al. Endemic mycoses in patients with STAT3-mutated hyper-IgE (Job) syndrome. J Allergy Clin Immunol 2015;136(5):1411–3.e1-2.
13. Siegel AM, Heimall J, Freeman AF, et al. A critical role for STAT3 transcription factor signaling in the development and maintenance of human T cell memory. Immunity 2011;35(5):806–18.
14. Hox V, O'Connell MP, Lyons JJ, et al. Diminution of signal transducer and activator of transcription 3 signaling inhibits vascular permeability and anaphylaxis. J Allergy Clin Immunol 2016;138(1):187–99.
15. Kumanovics A, Perkins SL, Gilbert H, et al. Diffuse large B cell lymphoma in hyper-IgE syndrome due to STAT3 mutation. J Clin Immunol 2010;30(6):886–93.
16. Leonard GD, Posadas E, Herrmann PC, et al. Non-Hodgkin's lymphoma in Job's syndrome: a case report and literature review. Leuk Lymphoma 2004;45(12):2521–5.
17. Grimbacher B, Holland SM, Gallin JI, et al. Hyper-IgE syndrome with recurrent infections–an autosomal dominant multisystem disorder. N Engl J Med 1999;340(9):692–702.
18. O'Connell AC, Puck JM, Grimbacher B, et al. Delayed eruption of permanent teeth in hyperimmunoglobulinemia E recurrent infection syndrome. Oral Surg Oral Med Oral Pathol Oral Radiol Endod 2000;89(2):177–85.
19. Domingo DL, Freeman AF, Davis J, et al. Novel intraoral phenotypes in hyperimmunoglobulin-E syndrome. Oral Dis 2008;14(1):73–81.
20. Freeman AF, Avila EM, Shaw PA, et al. Coronary artery abnormalities in Hyper-IgE syndrome. J Clin Immunol 2011;31(3):338–45.
21. Abd-Elmoniem KZ, Ramos N, Yazdani SK, et al. Coronary atherosclerosis and dilation in hyper IgE syndrome patients: depiction by magnetic resonance vessel wall imaging and pathological correlation. Atherosclerosis 2017;258:20–5.
22. Freeman AF, Collura-Burke CJ, Patronas NJ, et al. Brain abnormalities in patients with hyperimmunoglobulin E syndrome. Pediatrics 2007;119(5):e1121–5.
23. Sowerwine KJ, Holland SM, Freeman AF. Hyper-IgE syndrome update. Ann N Y Acad Sci 2012;1250:25–32.
24. Arora M, Bagi P, Strongin A, et al. Gastrointestinal manifestations of STAT3-deficient Hyper-IgE syndrome. J Clin Immunol 2017;37(7):695–700.
25. Milner JD, Brenchley JM, Laurence A, et al. Impaired T(H)17 cell differentiation in subjects with autosomal dominant hyper-IgE syndrome. Nature 2008;452(7188):773–6.
26. Takeda K, Noguchi K, Shi W, et al. Targeted disruption of the mouse Stat3 gene leads to early embryonic lethality. Proc Natl Acad Sci U S A 1997;94(8):3801–4.

27. Heimall J, Davis J, Shaw PA, et al. Paucity of genotype-phenotype correlations in STAT3 mutation positive Hyper IgE Syndrome (HIES). Clin Immunol 2011;139(1): 75–84.

28. Nieminen P, Morgan NV, Fenwick AL, et al. Inactivation of IL11 signaling causes craniosynostosis, delayed tooth eruption, and supernumerary teeth. Am J Hum Genet 2011;89(1):67–81.

29. Sekhsaria V, Dodd LE, Hsu AP, et al. Plasma metalloproteinase levels are dysregulated in signal transducer and activator of transcription 3 mutated hyper-IgE syndrome. J Allergy Clin Immunol 2011;128(5):1124–7.

30. Chandesris MO, Melki I, Natividad A, et al. Autosomal dominant STAT3 deficiency and hyper-IgE syndrome: molecular, cellular, and clinical features from a French national survey. Medicine (Baltimore) 2012;91(4):e1–19.

31. Nester TA, Wagnon AH, Reilly WF, et al. Effects of allogeneic peripheral stem cell transplantation in a patient with job syndrome of hyperimmunoglobulinemia E and recurrent infections. Am J Med 1998;105(2):162–4.

32. Gennery AR, Flood TJ, Abinun M, et al. Bone marrow transplantation does not correct the hyper IgE syndrome. Bone Marrow Transplant 2000;25(12):1303–5.

33. Goussetis E, Peristeri I, Kitra V, et al. Successful long-term immunologic reconstitution by allogeneic hematopoietic stem cell transplantation cures patients with autosomal dominant hyper-IgE syndrome. J Allergy Clin Immunol 2010;126(2): 392–4.

34. Greil J, Rausch T, Giese T, et al. Whole-exome sequencing links caspase recruitment domain 11 (CARD11) inactivation to severe combined immunodeficiency. J Allergy Clin Immunol 2013;131(5):1376–83.e3.

35. Snow AL, Xiao W, Stinson JR, et al. Congenital B cell lymphocytosis explained by novel germline CARD11 mutations. J Exp Med 2012;209(12):2247–61.

36. Renner ED, Puck JM, Holland SM, et al. Autosomal recessive hyperimmunoglobulin E syndrome: a distinct disease entity. J Pediatr 2004;144(1):93–9.

37. Aydin SE, Kilic SS, Aytekin C, et al. DOCK8 deficiency: clinical and immunological phenotype and treatment options - a review of 136 patients. J Clin Immunol 2015;35(2):189–98.

38. Engelhardt KR, Gertz ME, Keles S, et al. The extended clinical phenotype of 64 patients with dedicator of cytokinesis 8 deficiency. J Allergy Clin Immunol 2015; 136(2):402–12.

39. Al-Herz W, Ragupathy R, Massaad MJ, et al. Clinical, immunologic and genetic profiles of DOCK8-deficient patients in Kuwait. Clin Immunol 2012;143(3):266–72.

40. Shah NN, Freeman AF, Parta M, et al. Haploidentical transplantation for DOCK8 deficiency. Blood 2015;126(23):2229.

41. Dimitrova D, Freeman AF. Current status of dedicator of cytokinesis-associated immunodeficiency: DOCK8 and DOCK2. Dermatol Clin 2017;35(1):11–9.

42. Caracciolo S, Moratto D, Giacomelli M, et al. Expansion of CCR4+ activated T cells is associated with memory B cell reduction in DOCK8-deficient patients. Clin Immunol 2014;152(1–2):164–70.

43. Randall KL, Chan SS, Ma CS, et al. DOCK8 deficiency impairs CD8 T cell survival and function in humans and mice. J Exp Med 2011;208(11):2305–20.

44. Al-Zahrani D, Raddadi A, Massaad M, et al. Successful interferon-alpha 2b therapy for unremitting warts in a patient with DOCK8 deficiency. Clin Immunol 2014; 153(1):104–8.

45. Keles S, Jabara HH, Reisli I, et al. Plasmacytoid dendritic cell depletion in DOCK8 deficiency: rescue of severe herpetic infections with IFN-alpha 2b therapy. J Allergy Clin Immunol 2014;133(6):1753–5.e3.

46. McGhee SA, Chatila TA. DOCK8 immune deficiency as a model for primary cyto-skeletal dysfunction. Dis Markers 2010;29(3–4):151–6.
47. Ham H, Guerrier S, Kim J, et al. Dedicator of cytokinesis 8 interacts with talin and Wiskott-Aldrich syndrome protein to regulate NK cell cytotoxicity. J Immunol 2013;190(7):3661–9.
48. Zhang Q, Dove CG, Hor JL, et al. DOCK8 regulates lymphocyte shape integrity for skin antiviral immunity. J Exp Med 2014;211(13):2549–66.
49. Randall KL, Lambe T, Johnson AL, et al. Dock8 mutations cripple B cell immuno-logical synapses, germinal centers and long-lived antibody production. Nat Im-munol 2009;10(12):1283–91.
50. Jabara HH, McDonald DR, Janssen E, et al. DOCK8 functions as an adaptor that links TLR-MyD88 signaling to B cell activation. Nat Immunol 2012;13(6):612–20.
51. Sun X, Wang J, Qin T, et al. Dock8 regulates BCR signaling and activation of memory B cells via WASP and CD19. Blood Adv 2018;2(4):401–13.
52. Sassi A, Lazaroski S, Wu G, et al. Hypomorphic homozygous mutations in phos-phoglucomutase 3 (*PGM3*) impair immunity and increase serum IgE levels. J Allergy Clin Immunol 2014;133(5):1410–9, 1419.e1-3.
53. Stray-Pedersen A, Backe PH, Sorte HS, et al. *PGM3* mutations cause a congen-ital disorder of glycosylation with severe immunodeficiency and skeletal dysplasia. Am J Hum Genet 2014;95(1):96–107.
54. Bernth-Jensen JM, Holm M, Christiansen M. Neonatal-onset T(-)B(-)NK(+) severe combined immunodeficiency and neutropenia caused by mutated phosphoglu-comutase 3. J Allergy Clin Immunol 2016;137(1):321–4.
55. Pacheco-Cuellar G, Gauthier J, Desilets V, et al. A novel *PGM3* mutation is asso-ciated with a severe phenotype of bone marrow failure, severe combined immu-nodeficiency, skeletal dysplasia, and congenital malformations. J Bone Miner Res 2017;32(9):1853–9.
56. Lyons JJ, Milner JD, Rosenzweig SD. Glycans instructing immunity: the emerging role of altered glycosylation in clinical immunology. Front Pediatr 2015;3:54.

Early-Onset Inflammatory Bowel Disease

Judith R. Kelsen, MD[a], Pierre Russo, MD[b], Kathleen E. Sullivan, MD, PhD[c],*

KEYWORDS

- VEO-IBD • Primary immunodeficiencies • Inflammation • Monogenic

KEY POINTS

- The epidemiology of inflammatory bowel disease (IBD) is changing with increased incidence and a younger age of onset recently.
- Approximately 20% of the very early onset IBD cohorts have an inherited primary immunodeficiency.
- The evaluation of patients can use a multimodal approach, but ultimately often relies on genetic sequencing.

INTRODUCTION

Inflammatory bowel disease (IBD) is a complex disorder associated with a dysregulated immune response to environmental triggers in the genetically susceptible host. The frequency of this condition is increasing dramatically around the world, with the greatest increases in developing countries and young children.[1–3] The etiopathogenesis of the disorder is understood very poorly and the reasons for the increase in frequency in industrialized countries are probably multifactorial. Proposed mechanisms driving the increased incidence of IBD include increased antibiotic use, decreasing exposure to parasites and other infections, changes in diet, including the adoption of prepared foods that include emulsifiers and surfactants, all of which contribute to alterations in the gut microbiome.[4] Although IBD in young children has always been uncommon,

Disclosure Statement: The authors would like to acknowledge support from The Children's Hospital of Philadelphia, the Wallace Chair of Pediatrics, and K23 DK100461.

The US Immunodeficiency Network (USIDNET) data were supplied by the following contributors who provided at least 1% of the data for analysis: Ramsay Fuleihan, Elizabeth Garabedian, Charlotte Cunningham-Rundles, Rebecca Marsh, Hans D. Ochs, Avni Joshi, Daniel Suez, Elizabeth A. Secord, John Routes, Javeed Akhter, Francisco A. Bonilla, Jennifer Puck, Niraj Patel, Rebecca Buckley, Patricia Lugar, Burcin Uygungil, Gary Kleiner, and Morton J. Cowan.

[a] Division of Gastroenterology, Hepatology and Nutrition, 3401 Civic Center Boulevard, Philadelphia, PA 19104, USA; [b] Department of Pathology, Division of Allergy Immunology, The Children's Hospital of Philadelphia, ARC 1216-I, 3615 Civic Center Boulevard, Philadelphia, PA 19104, USA; [c] Division of Allergy Immunology, The Children's Hospital of Philadelphia, 3615 Civic Center Boulevard, Philadelphia, PA 19104, USA
* Corresponding author.
E-mail address: sullivank@email.chop.edu

Immunol Allergy Clin N Am 39 (2019) 63–79
https://doi.org/10.1016/j.iac.2018.08.008
0889-8561/19/© 2018 Elsevier Inc. All rights reserved.

this group is now experiencing the greatest increase in incidence.[3] In previous years, immunologists called on to see a very young child with IBD could be nearly certain that there would be an immunodeficiency. Today, with the rising incidence, it is more difficult to identify children with an inborn error of immunity who are presenting with IBD versus those children who have more typical polygenic inheritance with an exceptionally early onset of disease. This group of children with early-onset IBD, regardless of whether there is an inborn error of immunity, suffers from very high morbidity and a high burden of disease. This review is focused on understanding the immunologic contributors to IBD, the epidemiology, and the role of the immunologist in the diagnosis and management of patients with very early onset IBD (VEO-IBD).

The gastrointestinal tract is the largest immune organ in the body. Thus, it is no surprise that people with known immune deficiencies are at increased risk of developing IBD (**Fig. 1**). Classic IBD, as well as autoimmune enteropathy occur with high frequency in children with inborn errors of immunity, and studies have demonstrated that patients with significant enteropathy both have a shortened life expectancy and profoundly worse quality of life in common variable immunodeficiency.[5] There are clues to the immunologic underpinning of polygenic IBD from genome-wide association studies (GWAS). There is a strong association between major histocompatibility complex (MHC) haplotypes and IBD across multiple large GWAS.[6–8] Additional genes implicated in these large studies include those relevant for immunologic function as well as those related to barrier function of the gastrointestinal tract.[9] Other evidence supporting a key immunologic role in all types of IBD include gene expression arrays that demonstrate disordered function of the immune system.[10,11] This review focuses on those children with inborn errors of immunity that drive the development of VEO-IBD. These children provide key insights into the mechanisms of disease in IBD. Our understanding today of who develops IBD, why they develop IBD, and which type of therapy is most likely to yield the perfect balance between control of disease and minimizing adverse events is clearly better than in the past; however, it remains

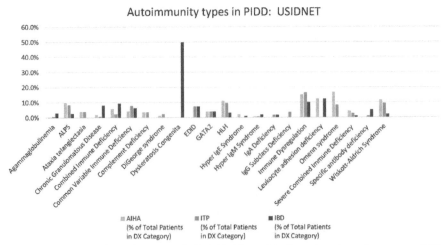

Fig. 1. Autoimmune hemolytic anemia (AIHA), idiopathic thrombocytopenia purpura (ITP), and IBD frequencies in different primary immunodeficiencies (PIDDs). US Immunodeficiency Network (USIDNET) data were extracted and graphed to display the frequencies of the 3 different types of autoimmune diseases. ALPS, autoimmune lymphoproliferative syndrome; EDID, ectodermal dysplasia immunodeficiency; HLH, hemophagocytic lymphohistiocytosis.

remarkably difficult to counsel families regarding prognosis when the onset of IBD is early in life. It is worth reflecting on the progress we have made in understanding inflammation to provide context for our current understanding of IBD.

THE ANCIENT UNDERSTANDING OF INFLAMMATION

Hippocrates believed that inflammation was integral to healing and introduced the word edema to the medical community. Indeed, inflammation leads to secretion of angiogenic and fibroblast growth factors regulating healing.[12] Thus, inflammation is not intrinsically deleterious. It serves a key role in host defense and promotes healing in physiologic settings. The key concepts of inflammation were first articulated by Aulus Celsus, 500 years after Hippocrates, when redness, warmth, swelling, and pain were articulated as manifestations of inflammation. Vasodilation accounts for the redness and warmth associated with inflammation and vascular leak accounts for the swelling or edema. When Antony van Leeuwenhoek improved the lens sufficiently to see individual cells, one of his first targets was to describe microcirculation changes related to inflammation. Dutrochet saw that white cells accumulate in inflammation in 1824. These studies paved the way to consider an integrated view of circulation as a pipeline for white cell delivery. Thus, the ancient understanding of inflammation evolved to a basic mechanistic understanding by the mid-1800s. Still today, we use the character of the invading cells to define the type of inflammation we seek to treat.

If inflammation represents an ancient concept that has been refined over the years, autoimmunity represents a much more recent concept. The overall concept of immunity sputtered through history, beginning with Thucydides' description of the plague of Athens rendering sufferers immune to a second attack. In 1900, Paul Ehrlich stated flatly that antibodies could not be generated to self, and it was only in the 1950s that autoantibodies were clearly demonstrated in human disease states. IBD is traditionally described as an inflammatory disease; however, therapy with T-cell–directed agents has achieved new prominence, supporting a model in which IBD is driven by true autoimmunity.

Today, we continue to characterize the inflammatory cell infiltrate as a strategy to inform on our understanding (see later in this article). The most common biologic therapy, use of a tumor necrosis factor (TNF) inhibitor, is predicated on the common observation that neutrophils are the most common infiltrating cell type in colitis and that inhibition of TNF diminishes their migration out of the vascular space and into the tissue.[13] We treat the general elements of inflammation using aspirin derivatives that dampen leukotriene and prostaglandin pathways, a concept that Celsus described and was exploited by Imhotep in ancient Egypt using willow bark.[14,15]

TYPES OF INFLAMMATORY BOWEL DISEASE

Textbooks often emphasize the distinction between Crohn disease and ulcerative colitis. Indeed, there are important clinical differences. The key differences are highlighted in **Table 1**. Crohn disease is characterized by transmural pleomorphic inflammation and the deep involvement leads to fistulas and abscesses. Granulomas are often seen and any part of the intestine can be involved. In addition, Crohn disease can involve the entire gastrointestinal tract, including perianal disease. In ulcerative colitis, the inflammation is limited to the colon and is most often characterized by a neutrophilic inflammation. Both can be associated with extraintestinal features and both have significant complications. Gene expression arrays have identified differences and commonalities in the 2 types of IBD.[11,16–18] Indeterminate IBD or

Table 1
Comparison of Crohn disease and ulcerative colitis

Feature	Crohn Disease	Ulcerative Colitis
Typical site of initiation	Terminal ileum	Rectum
Pattern	Skip lesions	Extends proximally
Layers affected	Transmural	Submucosa/mucosa
Pathology	Granulomas, fissures	Crypt abscesses, pseudopolyps
Complications	Fistulas, abscess	Hemorrhage, toxic megacolon
Risk of colon cancer	+	++
Extraintestinal symptoms	Fever, arthritis, pyoderma gangrenosa, Sweet syndrome	Hepatitis, sclerosing cholangitis, pyoderma gangrenosa, Sweet syndrome, arthritis

IBD-undifferentiated (IBD-U) are terms used to classify patients with clear evidence of IBD but for whom neither Crohn disease nor ulcerative colitis can be confidently diagnosed. This class is much more common in children than in adults, in whom 5% to 10% of patients with IBD are initially classified as IBD-U.[19] This is particularly so for the very young children, with onset at younger than 6 years of age, known as VEO-IBD. These children can present with pancolonic disease, but over time, disease can extend to other locations.[20–23]

Pathologic Features of Inflammatory Bowel Disease and Very Early Onset Inflammatory Bowel Disease

There are several compelling reasons to perform endoscopy/colonoscopy in the setting of IBD or suspected IBD[24]:

- Establishing or confirming the diagnosis of IBD
- Distinguishing between Crohn disease and ulcerative colitis
- Defining the extent of inflammation (critical for therapy)
- Evaluating for dysplasia or malignancy
- Monitoring efficacy of therapy

The pathologic findings may be divided by anatomic location or structural derivation and it is useful to partition the evaluation in this way. Pathology reports may use the PAID reporting system of Pattern, Activity, Interpretation, and Dysplasia and typically report the follow features:

- Architectural features: crypt structure, surface irregularity, villi in the small bowel
- Inflammatory features: neutrophils, lymphocytes, granulomas
- Epithelial: Paneth cell metaplasia, mucin depletion

The normal colon is characterized by beautiful regular crypts (**Fig. 2**). The crypts extend from the luminal surface to the muscularis layer in regular parallel columns. Plasma cells are common in the upper third, but are infrequent or absent near the muscularis mucosa. In the cecum and ascending colon, more plasma cells are seen and they may be found throughout the lamina propria.[24] Acute inflammation is described when cryptitis, crypt abscesses, and/or ulceration are seen. To diagnose IBD, chronic changes also must be observed. These include crypt distortion, crypt branching (rare branched crypts on an otherwise normal sample are acceptable), crypt atrophy, and basal plasma cell expansion (**Fig. 3**). Granulomas are also classified as chronic changes. Additional features of chronic changes include Paneth cell metaplasia with

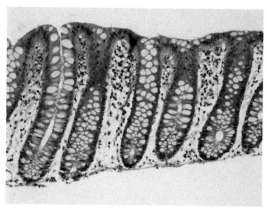

Fig. 2. Normal colonic architecture with regular crypts. Clear goblet cells in the crypts are abundant. There are few cells between the crypts. Hematoxylin and eosin stain. Original magnification ×200.

eosinophilic inclusions and mucin depletion. This latter finding is highly subjective but refers to the goblet cell mucin that is normally abundant in crypts. The time course of these chronic changes varies, but most are observed within a few months of onset.[25] Nevertheless, it is not uncommon to observe acute changes without chronic features when biopsies are performed near the disease onset. In this setting, IBD cannot be diagnosed.[26] Although chronic changes can be detected shortly after onset of symptoms, or even prior, many patients have had symptoms for several months before seeking medical attention. Thus, this practical consideration is relevant in a minority of patients.

The pathologic features more characteristic of VEO-IBD compared with older pediatric and adult-onset IBD include eosinophils in the crypts and apoptotic crypt cells (**Fig. 4**). These are seldom seen in adult IBD unless the disease is very active but are common in VEO-IBD. The finding of eosinophils can cause confusion with allergy or eosinophilic gastroenteridites.[27] When apoptotic cells are abundant, the pathology may resemble graft versus host disease and can be associated with dyskeratosis congenita.[28]

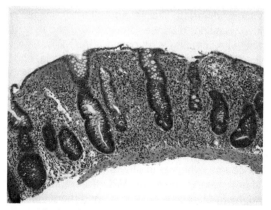

Fig. 3. Shortened crypts with abundant inflammation in the lamina propria in a 2-year-old child with IBD. Crypts are irregular and goblet cells are diminished. Hematoxylin and eosin stain. Original magnification ×100.

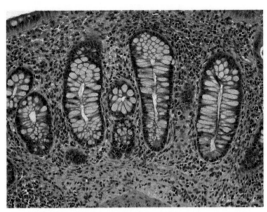

Fig. 4. IBD in a 5-year-old child demonstrating an intense eosinophilic infiltrate in the lamina propria. Hematoxylin and eosin stain. Original magnification ×200.

Involvement of the small bowel is less well characterized in VEO-IBD but villous atrophy can be a feature. Small bowel involvement is not uncommon in Crohn disease and the pattern is a mixed inflammatory cell infiltrate. Villous blunting or atrophy is uncommon in adult IBD cohorts but is seen in as many as 20% of the VEO-IBD cohort.

DIFFERENTIAL DIAGNOSIS OF INFLAMMATORY BOWEL DISEASE

There are 2 main considerations in a previously well child, although the entire differential is considerable (**Table 2**). Infection is more common statistically in this age range than IBD. Tuberculosis, amebiasis, *Clostridium difficile*, cryptosporidia, and schistosomiasis have distinctive pathologic features recognizable on endoscopy. The most common issue is distinguishing acute infection with *Campylobacter*, *C difficile* colitis, *Salmonella*, or *Shigella* from acute onset of IBD in childhood.[25,29,30] Cryptitis and crypt abscesses may be features of infectious colitis (**Fig. 5**). Basal plasmacytosis and abnormal crypt architecture strongly favor inflammation due to infectious causes.[24,31] In adults and older children, there are several mimics of IBD that should be considered but they are seldom relevant for the VEO-IBD population (see **Table 2**). The second consideration is food protein–induced enterocolitis (FPIES). Both conditions can present abruptly with bloody diarrhea. Classic acute FPIES usually occurs in an infant who exhibits repetitive vomiting, diarrhea, dehydration, and hypovolemic shock.[32,33] The very acute setting with vomiting is atypical for VEO-IBD. Of more concern is the rare entity of chronic FPIES in which chronic diarrhea, anemia, and hypoalbuminemia may be seen.[34] This is very typical for VEO-IBD and an additional confusion is the finding of tissue eosinophilia in both on biopsy. Chronic crypt changes are not common in FPIES; however, there are limited data on the pathologic features of chronic FPIES.[35]

CLINICAL FEATURES OF VERY EARLY ONSET INFLAMMATORY BOWEL DISEASE

Early-onset disease in many conditions such as systemic lupus erythematosus portends a more difficult course, whereas in others, such as Henoch Schönlein purpura, children fare better than adults. Patients with VEO-IBD, regardless of whether a monogenic cause is found, have more severe disease and more years of disease burden. Thus, they accrue damage disproportionately. Some metrics of disease severity include the higher rate of surgical intervention, higher rate of extraintestinal manifestations, and higher failure rate of TNF inhibitors. Children also exhibit growth failure

Table 2
Differential diagnosis of colitis with chronic changes on pathology

Consideration	Notes
Diversion proctocolitis	The excluded large bowel can show changes similar to IBD
Microscopic colitis (collagenous colitis or lymphocytic colitis)	These are not uncommon in primary immunodeficiency disorders but respond to alternative therapies
Diverticular colitis	Sigmoid disease usually in older adults with diverticulitis
Radiation colitis	Fibrosis and vascular changes are characteristic in addition to chronic inflammation
Ischemic colitis	The anatomic distribution is distinctive although the pathologic appearance can resemble IBD
Graft vs host disease	Pathologically is nearly indistinguishable from IBD, although apoptotic crypt epithelial cells are prominent
HIV-related colitis	HIV testing and extensive pathogen testing required
Lymphogranuloma venereum	Testing for syphilis can diagnose this, which is typically seen in the setting of HIV
Yersinia	Abundant granulomas with central necrosis
Tuberculosis	Large granulomas
Nonsteroidal anti-inflammatory use	Epithelial cell apoptosis prominent
Mycophenolate mofetil	Pathology indistinguishable from IBD
Behcet disease	Lymphoid aggregates
Autoimmune enteropathy	Distinct autoantibodies; common in primary immunodeficiencies

Abbreviations: HIV, human immunodeficiency virus; IBD, inflammatory bowel disease.

probably in part due to compromised nutrition and in part due to chronic inflammation. Less commonly, chronic corticosteroids may play a role. The disease is more likely to be colonic in VEO-IBD compared with older children and adults. This is notable because some of the monogenic causes are associated with panenteric disease.

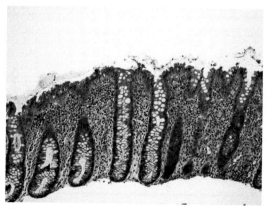

Fig. 5. Bacterial gastroenteritis demonstrates normal crypt architecture and inflammation that is more pronounced at the luminal surface. Hematoxylin and eosin stain. Original magnification ×100.

The extraintestinal features can drive the selection of therapy. As an example, the treatment in cases with sclerosing cholangitis, thought to be due to a T-cell–driven process, often uses corticosteroids, azathioprine, cyclosporine, or tacrolimus. Extraintestinal features differ somewhat between Crohn disease and ulcerative colitis in adults. The only available data have been collected in adults (**Table 3**). These features also are highly influenced by MHC alleles.[36] Arthritis and spondyloarthropathy occur more frequently in children than adults, but there has been little effort to compare these manifestations in head-to-head comparisons of children and adults (**Table 4**).[37–39]

Genetics of Inflammatory Bowel Disease

IBD has long been recognized as having a heritable component. It is found at higher rates in Caucasian individuals, especially those with Jewish ancestry.[40] The relative risk for a sibling of a patient with IBD is 13 to 26 for Crohn disease and 7 to 17 for ulcerative colitis.[41] Monozygotic twin concordance rates are 30% for Crohn disease and 15% for ulcerative colitis.[42–44] When GWASs have been performed, the MHC class II region has had a strong signal, implicating T cells in the pathophysiology.[45] NOD2 (also known as CARD11) was one of the first variants to exhibit a strong association with IBD.[46] The effect is limited to Crohn disease. The 3 common variants (R702W, G908R, L1007fs) all impair activation of the NOD2 signaling pathway by its biological ligand, muramyl dipeptide.[47] These variants can therefore be considered to represent an immunodeficiency related to innate pattern recognition. A single NOD2 risk allele confers a relative risk of 2-fold to 3-fold over the general population, whereas 2 risk alleles confer a relative risk of 17-fold.[48,49] Additional genes identified by GWASs have strongly implicated the immune system in the pathogenesis of IBD.[50] Cytokine pathways and autophagy gene variants have been prominent findings.[51,52] Not all loci identified in adult studies have been found in pediatric studies and vice versa; however, the pathways identified appear comparable.[53–57] When whole-exome sequencing has been performed, enrichment in rare variants related to immune function have been identified.[58,59] Interestingly, most of the genes implicated in the GWASs of IBD have been implicated in various other autoimmune diseases both in children and adults.[60] These data suggest that compromised tolerance or immune function can impact susceptibility to autoimmunity in a general way, with the specific phenotype manifested differentially depending on environment or other genes.

IBD has been long recognized as associated with primary immunodeficiencies. In some cases, the association is very high, as for IKBKG (NF-kappa-B essential

Table 3
Extraintestinal manifestations in adults

Finding	Crohn Disease, %	Ulcerative Colitis, %
Erythema nodosum	6	3
Pyoderma gangrenosum	2	2
Skin tags	37	Low
Orofacial granulomatosis	<1	Low
Oral ulcers	10	4
Large joint arthritis	15	8
Spondyloarthropathy	6	2
Uveitis	6	4
Sclerosing cholangitis	<1	3
Nephrolithiasis	5	5

Table 4
Extraintestinal manifestations in adults and children

Finding	Children, %	Adults, %
Growth failure	30	—
Erythema nodosum	4	2
Pyoderma gangrenosum	2	1
Oral ulcers	7	7.5
Arthritis	20	7
Spondyloarthropathy	5	1
Uveitis	4	2
Sclerosing cholangitis	2	1

modulator [NEMO]), CYBB (chronic granulomatous disease [CGD]), and BTK (agammaglobulinemia [XLA]) deficiencies, whereas in other gene defects only a single or a few cases of IBD have been reported. In common variable immune deficiency (CVID), various autoimmune diseases, including IBD, are fairly common (see **Fig. 1**). Most other primary immunodeficiencies, however, are enriched for a single prominent type of autoimmune disease. Mechanisms are infrequently fully understood even in these settings with a single-gene effect. Altered signaling leading to compromised tolerance are invoked for many disorders that primarily impact lymphocyte function, whereas impaired surveillance of the enteric surface is often invoked related to innate immune defects, such as CGD.[61,62] In all cases, an altered microbiome is likely to contribute to IBD susceptibility.[63]

A common conundrum for clinical immunologists is to determine which among the growing cohort of young children with IBD have an underlying primary immunodeficiency. The question is not simply academic. Although therapy for some patients with VEO-IBD can be straightforward, treatment can be difficult and subject to frequent failure.[64–66] The therapy for those with primary immunodeficiencies can be even more difficult.[67,68] Knowing the gene defect can be extremely helpful in defining the therapy (**Table 5**).

Table 5
Unique therapeutic options in patients with IBD due to monogenic primary immunodeficiencies

Gene Defect	Therapeutic Considerations
XIAP (X-linked lymphoproliferative disease)	HSCT, IL-18 binding protein study under way
CYBB and other etiologies of CGD	IL-1 blockade; TNF inhibitors should not be used due to risk of fungal infections
IL10, IL10RA, IL10RB	HSCT
TTC7A	HSCT can be considered; however, success has been limited
LRBA	Abatacept, sirolimus, colchicine, HSCT
CTLA4	Abatacept, sirolimus, HSCT
MEFV (Familial Mediterranean Fever)	IL-1 blockade, colchicine
NLRC4	IL-18 binding protein

Abbreviations: HSCT, hematopoietic stem cell transplantation; IL, interleukin; TNF, tumor necrosis factor.

There is no single biomarker that cleanly segregates patients having an underlying immunodeficiency from those who do not. Instead, it is useful to think of red flags for the consideration for sequencing, which is the most ensured way to establish a diagnosis.[68,69] Infantile onset is always a concern for a monogenic cause. In a key finding reported by Uhlig and colleagues,[68] the earlier the onset of IBD, the more likely that there was a monogenic cause. All the patients they reported with interleukin (IL)-10 pathway, TTC7A, PLCG2, and ADAM17 defects had onset of IBD in infancy. Atypical severe combined immunodeficiency (SCID), severe dyskeratosis congenita, and IPEX cases developed IBD in childhood. These contrast with Wiskott-Aldrich syndrome, CGD, LRBA (CVID phenotype), IKBKG (NEMO), XIAP, Hermansky Pudlak syndrome, and other B-cell defects that had a very broad spread in age of onset, with some cases developing IBD in adulthood. The impact of this study cannot be overstated. Patients with primary immunodeficiencies are usually identified before adulthood, but the important implication of this study is that for many single-gene defects, presentation could even occur in adulthood. Indeed, studies of adult cohorts have uniformly revealed monogenic cases at a low rate.[70–73] Age of onset is useful, therefore, in risk-stratifying, but there is age cutoff after which the concern for a monogenic cause is no longer valid.

If age is imperfect, what other features are useful? The pathology is another example of a useful yet imperfect predictor of a monogenic cause. Panenteric disease, villous blunting, tissue eosinophilia, and increased epithelial apoptosis are other useful data points that suggest a monogenic cause. Finally, flow cytometry is not useful in the IL-10 family of defects but can provide some supportive evidence in other cases. For the typical lymphocyte defects, inverted CD4/CD8, low T-cell counts, absent B cells, and other key findings may point to a cause. A dihydrorhodamine test for CGD should always be performed because TNF inhibitors are contraindicated in CGD.[74]

Finally, the clinical history and family history are very helpful in many cases. Although a positive family history is common in IBD and VEO-IBD, a family history of other conditions may point toward a single unifying explanation. The clinical history may exhibit classic infectious signs to suggest an immunodeficiency, but that is not very typical. The most helpful historic features are often other autoimmune diseases. Multiple severe autoimmune diseases support a monogenic cause. Hemophagocytic syndrome represents another notable clinical finding in the patient or in a sibling.

It may be appreciated that although we currently lack a single biomarker, armed with the knowledge of less common features that are predictive, judicious ordering of genetic testing can be pursued. Today, there are IBD gene panels and whole-exome sequencing that are reasonably cost-effective compared with the cost of continued complications and hospitalizations. **Table 6** lists monogenic causes of VEO-IBD. This list does not include single cases and it is important to recognize that the landscape changes very quickly.

A Strategy to Evaluate Patients with Very Early Onset Inflammatory Bowel Disease

There is no single appropriate approach to workup of children with VEO-IBD. The community must share experiences and develop an approach that is based on evidence. Many centers are developing a joint gastroenterology-immunology approach to this patient population. This will likely yield important insights. In this spirit, this article shares 1 approach to the evaluation.

Establishing the diagnosis of IBD:

- Rule out infection with stool culture, ova, and parasite examination
- Fecal calprotectin (this can be low in infants with IBD)
- Endoscopy and colonoscopy

Table 6
Monogenic causes of very early onset inflammatory bowel disease

Gene Name	Disease Name	Category
ADAM17		Barrier dysfunction
AICDA	Hyper IgM	Humoral
BTK	X-linked agammaglobulinemia	Humoral
CD40LG	X-linked Hyper IgM	Humoral
CTLA4		Humoral
CYBA	CGD	Neutrophil
CYBB	CGD	Neutrophil
DKC1	Dyskeratosis congenita	Telomeropathy
DOCK8		Combined immunodeficiency
FOXP3	IPEX	Immune dysregulation
HSP4	Hermansky Pudlak	Immune dysregulation
ICOS		Immune dysregulation
IKBKG	NEMO	Combined immunodeficiency
IL10		Immune dysregulation
IL10RA		Immune dysregulation
IL10RB		Immune dysregulation
IL21		Humoral
IL2RA		Combined immunodeficiency
IL2RB		Combined immunodeficiency
ITCH		Immune dysregulation
ITGB2	LAD1	Neurophil
LIG4		Combined immunodeficiency
LRBA		Immune dysregulation
MEFV	Familial Mediterranean fever	Immune dysregulation
MVK	Hyper IgD syndrome	Immune dysregulation
NCF2	CGD	Neutrophil
NCF4	CGD	Neutrophil
NFAT5		Immune dysregulation
NLRC4		Immune dysregulation
PIK3CD		Immune dysregulation
PIK3R1		Immune dysregulation
PLGC2		Immune dysregulation
RTEL1	Dyskeratosis congenita	Telomeropathy
SKIV2L	THE syndrome	Combined immunodeficiency
SLC7A4	Lysinuric protein intolerance	Immune dysregulation
STAT1 GOF		Immune dysregulation
STAT3 GOF		Immune dysregulation
STIM1		Combined immunodeficiency
STXBP2	HLH	Immune dysregulation
STXBP3	HLH	Immune dysregulation
TTC7A	Multiple intestinal atresia SCID	Combined immunodeficiency
TTC37	THE syndrome	Combined immunodeficiency

(continued on next page)

Table 6 (continued)		
Gene Name	**Disease Name**	**Category**
WAS	Wiskott-Aldrich syndrome	Combined immunodeficiency
XIAP	XLP2	Immune dysregulation

Exclusive of leaky severe combined immunodeficiency (SCID) and genetic causes of dyskeratosis congenita where inflammatory bowel disease has not been reported.

Abbreviations: CGD, chronic granulomatous disease; HLH, hemophagocytic lymphohistiocytosis; Ig, immunoglobulin; IPEX, immune dysregulation, polyendocrinopathy, X-linked syndrome; LAD, leukocyte adhesion deficiency; NEMO, NF-kappa-B essential modulator; THE, trichohepatic enteric; XLP, X-linked lymphoproliferative syndrome.

IBD in children with onset at age younger than 6 years: diagnostic evaluation for primary immunodeficiencies:

- Family history and clinical features: infections, autoimmunity, complications
- Review pathology to identify atypical features
- Dihydrorhodamine test for CGD
- Flow cytometry to assess T/B-cell subsets and maturation
- Consider:
  - Natural killer cell function
  - IL-10 suppression assay (identifies only IL-10 receptor defects)
  - Sequencing:
    - Currently, whole-exome sequencing offers the greatest sensitivity when paired with copy number variation
    - Many IBD sequencing panels are now offered and represent a strategy more likely to get insurance approval

Management approaches in VEO-IBD:

- Enteral nutrition
- Aminosalicylate derivatives (Azo-based formulations, such as balsalazide, act only in the colon; mesalamine formulations, such as Pentasa and Asacol, act in the terminal ileum and colon)
- Antibiotic treatment
- Probiotics
- Systemic corticosteroids (acutely)
- Topical steroids: budesonide (ileal release and rectal suppositories)
- 6-mercaptopurine and azathioprine (monitor for idiosyncratic reactions, seldom used in children due to risk of malignancy)
- Methotrexate (monitoring required, folate needed at higher doses)
- TNF inhibitors (contraindicated in CGD)
- Ustekinumab
- Tofacitinib (limited data)
- Vedolizumab
- Surgical diversion, colectomy
- Alternative options for refractory disease
  - IL-1 blockade
  - Rituximab
  - Cyclosporine
  - Tacrolimus
  - Sirolimus

SUMMARY

The landscape of VEO-IBD is changing in Westernized countries with decreasing age of incidence and increasing global frequency.[3] For clinical immunologists, this poses a difficult conundrum. There are imperfect strategies outside of sequencing to identify patients who have VEO-IBD due to a primary immunodeficiency. Clinical features, pathologic features, and flow cytometry can define a group at higher risk for a monogenic primary immunodeficiency, but to date there is no single biomarker. Sequencing options are almost bewildering, with multiple single-gene options, gene panels, and whole-exome sequencing. In our cohort, monogenic primary immunodeficiencies have been found in 20% of those with age of onset at younger than 6 years. Among those, novel genes have been identified at a frequency of 20% in the entire set of monogenic conditions. This suggests that gene panels, while useful, are also imperfect. Whole-exome approaches that filter out novel variants will miss a significant fraction of patients. Over time, with better data and collaborative approaches, the immunology/gastroenterology community will be able to more rationally design diagnostic approaches and direct development of gene panels appropriate for this population.

REFERENCES

1. Bach JF. The effect of infections on susceptibility to autoimmune and allergic diseases. N Engl J Med 2002;347(12):911–20.
2. Ng SC, Shi HY, Hamidi N, et al. Worldwide incidence and prevalence of inflammatory bowel disease in the 21st century: a systematic review of population-based studies. Lancet 2018;390(10114):2769–78.
3. Benchimol EI, Bernstein CN, Bitton A, et al. Trends in epidemiology of pediatric inflammatory bowel disease in Canada: distributed network analysis of multiple population-based provincial health administrative databases. Am J Gastroenterol 2017;112(7):1120–34.
4. Chassaing B, Koren O, Goodrich JK, et al. Dietary emulsifiers impact the mouse gut microbiota promoting colitis and metabolic syndrome. Nature 2015;519(7541): 92–6.
5. Chapel H, Lucas M, Lee M, et al. Common variable immunodeficiency disorders: division into distinct clinical phenotypes. Blood 2008;112(2):277–86.
6. Ahmad T, Marshall S, Jewell D. Genotype-based phenotyping heralds a new taxonomy for inflammatory bowel disease. Curr Opin Gastroenterol 2003;19(4): 327–35.
7. Stokkers PC, Reitsma PH, Tytgat GN, et al. HLA-DR and -DQ phenotypes in inflammatory bowel disease: a meta-analysis. Gut 1999;45(3):395–401.
8. Silverberg MS, Mirea L, Bull SB, et al. A population- and family-based study of Canadian families reveals association of HLA DRB1*0103 with colonic involvement in inflammatory bowel disease. Inflamm Bowel Dis 2003;9(1):1–9.
9. Peloquin JM, Goel G, Kong L, et al. Characterization of candidate genes in inflammatory bowel disease-associated risk loci. JCI Insight 2016;1(13):e87899.
10. Holgersen K, Kutlu B, Fox B, et al. High-resolution gene expression profiling using RNA sequencing in patients with inflammatory bowel disease and in mouse models of colitis. J Crohns Colitis 2015;9(6):492–506.
11. Costello CM, Mah N, Hasler R, et al. Dissection of the inflammatory bowel disease transcriptome using genome-wide cDNA microarrays. PLoS Med 2005;2(8):e199.
12. Koh TJ, DiPietro LA. Inflammation and wound healing: the role of the macrophage. Expert Rev Mol Med 2011;13:e23.

13. Silva LC, Ortigosa LC, Benard G. Anti-TNF-alpha agents in the treatment of immune-mediated inflammatory diseases: mechanisms of action and pitfalls. Immunotherapy 2010;2(6):817–33.

14. Lauritsen K, Laursen LS, Bukhave K, et al. Effects of topical 5-aminosalicylic acid and prednisolone on prostaglandin E2 and leukotriene B4 levels determined by equilibrium in vivo dialysis of rectum in relapsing ulcerative colitis. Gastroenterology 1986;91(4):837–44.

15. Mackowiak PA. Brief history of antipyretic therapy. Clin Infect Dis 2000;31(Suppl 5):S154–6.

16. Dieckgraefe BK, Stenson WF, Korzenik JR, et al. Analysis of mucosal gene expression in inflammatory bowel disease by parallel oligonucleotide arrays. Physiol Genomics 2000;4(1):1–11.

17. Lawrance IC, Fiocchi C, Chakravarti S. Ulcerative colitis and Crohn's disease: distinctive gene expression profiles and novel susceptibility candidate genes. Hum Mol Genet 2001;10(5):445–56.

18. Dooley TP, Curto EV, Reddy SP, et al. Regulation of gene expression in inflammatory bowel disease and correlation with IBD drugs: screening by DNA microarrays. Inflamm Bowel Dis 2004;10(1):1–14.

19. Geboes K, Van Eyken P. Inflammatory bowel disease unclassified and indeterminate colitis: the role of the pathologist. J Clin Pathol 2009;62(3):201–5.

20. Prenzel F, Uhlig HH. Frequency of indeterminate colitis in children and adults with IBD—a metaanalysis. J Crohns Colitis 2009;3(4):277–81.

21. Heyman MB, Kirschner BS, Gold BD, et al. Children with early-onset inflammatory bowel disease (IBD): analysis of a pediatric IBD consortium registry. J Pediatr 2005;146(1):35–40.

22. Carvalho RS, Abadom V, Dilworth HP, et al. Indeterminate colitis: a significant subgroup of pediatric IBD. Inflamm Bowel Dis 2006;12(4):258–62.

23. Henriksen M, Jahnsen J, Lygren I, et al. Change of diagnosis during the first five years after onset of inflammatory bowel disease: results of a prospective follow-up study (the IBSEN Study). Scand J Gastroenterol 2006;41(9):1037–43.

24. Feakins RM, British Society of G. Inflammatory bowel disease biopsies: updated British Society of Gastroenterology reporting guidelines. J Clin Pathol 2013; 66(12):1005–26.

25. Schumacher G, Kollberg B, Sandstedt B. A prospective study of first attacks of inflammatory bowel disease and infectious colitis. Histologic course during the 1st year after presentation. Scand J Gastroenterol 1994;29(4):318–32.

26. Tanaka M, Riddell RH, Saito H, et al. Morphologic criteria applicable to biopsy specimens for effective distinction of inflammatory bowel disease from other forms of colitis and of Crohn's disease from ulcerative colitis. Scand J Gastroenterol 1999;34(1):55–67.

27. Lowichik A, Weinberg AG. A quantitative evaluation of mucosal eosinophils in the pediatric gastrointestinal tract. Mod Pathol 1996;9(2):110–4.

28. Jyonouchi S, Forbes L, Ruchelli E, et al. Dyskeratosis congenita: a combined immunodeficiency with broad clinical spectrum—a single-center pediatric experience. Pediatr Allergy Immunol 2011;22(3):313–9.

29. Schumacher G, Sandstedt B, Kollberg B. A prospective study of first attacks of inflammatory bowel disease and infectious colitis. Clinical findings and early diagnosis. Scand J Gastroenterol 1994;29(3):265–74.

30. Surawicz CM, Belic L. Rectal biopsy helps to distinguish acute self-limited colitis from idiopathic inflammatory bowel disease. Gastroenterology 1984; 86(1):104–13.

31. Jenkins D, Goodall A, Scott BB. Simple objective criteria for diagnosis of causes of acute diarrhoea on rectal biopsy. J Clin Pathol 1997;50(7):580–5.
32. Sicherer SH. Food protein-induced enterocolitis syndrome: clinical perspectives. J Pediatr Gastroenterol Nutr 2000;30(Suppl):S45–9.
33. Leonard SA, Nowak-Wegrzyn A. Clinical diagnosis and management of food protein-induced enterocolitis syndrome. Curr Opin Pediatr 2012;24(6):739–45.
34. Mane SK, Bahna SL. Clinical manifestations of food protein-induced enterocolitis syndrome. Curr Opin Allergy Clin Immunol 2014;14(3):217–21.
35. Nowak-Wegrzyn A, Muraro A. Food protein-induced enterocolitis syndrome. Curr Opin Allergy Clin Immunol 2009;9(4):371–7.
36. Orchard TR, Chua CN, Ahmad T, et al. Uveitis and erythema nodosum in inflammatory bowel disease: clinical features and the role of HLA genes. Gastroenterology 2002;123(3):714–8.
37. Greuter T, Bertoldo F, Rechner R, et al. Extraintestinal manifestations of pediatric inflammatory bowel disease: prevalence, presentation, and anti-TNF treatment. J Pediatr Gastroenterol Nutr 2017;65(2):200–6.
38. Jose FA, Garnett EA, Vittinghoff E, et al. Development of extraintestinal manifestations in pediatric patients with inflammatory bowel disease. Inflamm Bowel Dis 2009;15(1):63–8.
39. Jose FA, Heyman MB. Extraintestinal manifestations of inflammatory bowel disease. J Pediatr Gastroenterol Nutr 2008;46(2):124–33.
40. Duerr RH. The genetics of inflammatory bowel disease. Gastroenterol Clin North Am 2002;31(1):63–76.
41. Laharie D, Debeugny S, Peeters M, et al. Inflammatory bowel disease in spouses and their offspring. Gastroenterology 2001;120(4):816–9.
42. Orholm M, Binder V, Sorensen TI, et al. Concordance of inflammatory bowel disease among Danish twins. Results of a nationwide study. Scand J Gastroenterol 2000;35(10):1075–81.
43. Thompson NP, Driscoll R, Pounder RE, et al. Genetics versus environment in inflammatory bowel disease: results of a British twin study. BMJ 1996;312(7023):95–6.
44. Tysk C, Lindberg E, Jarnerot G, et al. Ulcerative colitis and Crohn's disease in an unselected population of monozygotic and dizygotic twins. A study of heritability and the influence of smoking. Gut 1988;29(7):990–6.
45. Goyette P, Boucher G, Mallon D, et al. High-density mapping of the MHC identifies a shared role for HLA-DRB1*01:03 in inflammatory bowel diseases and heterozygous advantage in ulcerative colitis. Nat Genet 2015;47(2):172–9.
46. Lesage S, Zouali H, Cezard JP, et al. CARD15/NOD2 mutational analysis and genotype-phenotype correlation in 612 patients with inflammatory bowel disease. Am J Hum Genet 2002;70(4):845–57.
47. Li J, Moran T, Swanson E, et al. Regulation of IL-8 and IL-1beta expression in Crohn's disease associated NOD2/CARD15 mutations. Hum Mol Genet 2004;13(16):1715–25.
48. Economou M, Trikalinos TA, Loizou KT, et al. Differential effects of NOD2 variants on Crohn's disease risk and phenotype in diverse populations: a metaanalysis. Am J Gastroenterol 2004;99(12):2393–404.
49. Cummings JR, Jewell DP. Clinical implications of inflammatory bowel disease genetics on phenotype. Inflamm Bowel Dis 2005;11(1):56–61.
50. Duerr RH, Taylor KD, Brant SR, et al. A genome-wide association study identifies IL23R as an inflammatory bowel disease gene. Science 2006;314(5804):1461–3.

51. Hampe J, Franke A, Rosenstiel P, et al. A genome-wide association scan of non-synonymous SNPs identifies a susceptibility variant for Crohn disease in ATG16L1. Nat Genet 2007;39(2):207–11.
52. Rioux JD, Xavier RJ, Taylor KD, et al. Genome-wide association study identifies new susceptibility loci for Crohn disease and implicates autophagy in disease pathogenesis. Nat Genet 2007;39(5):596–604.
53. Levine A, Kugathasan S, Annese V, et al. Pediatric onset Crohn's colitis is characterized by genotype-dependent age-related susceptibility. Inflamm Bowel Dis 2007;13(12):1509–15.
54. Henderson P, van Limbergen JE, Wilson DC, et al. Genetics of childhood-onset inflammatory bowel disease. Inflamm Bowel Dis 2011;17(1):346–61.
55. Imielinski M, Baldassano RN, Griffiths A, et al. Common variants at five new loci associated with early-onset inflammatory bowel disease. Nat Genet 2009;41(12): 1335–40.
56. Kugathasan S, Baldassano RN, Bradfield JP, et al. Loci on 20q13 and 21q22 are associated with pediatric-onset inflammatory bowel disease. Nat Genet 2008; 40(10):1211–5.
57. Amre DK, Mack DR, Morgan K, et al. Investigation of reported associations between the 20q13 and 21q22 loci and pediatric-onset Crohn's disease in Canadian children. Am J Gastroenterol 2009;104(11):2824–8.
58. Ostrowski J, Paziewska A, Lazowska I, et al. Genetic architecture differences between pediatric and adult-onset inflammatory bowel diseases in the Polish population. Sci Rep 2016;6:39831.
59. Kelsen JR, Dawany N, Moran CJ, et al. Exome sequencing analysis reveals variants in primary immunodeficiency genes in patients with very early onset inflammatory bowel disease. Gastroenterology 2015;149(6):1415–24.
60. Zhernakova A, van Diemen CC, Wijmenga C. Detecting shared pathogenesis from the shared genetics of immune-related diseases. Nat Rev Genet 2009; 10(1):43–55.
61. Fischer A, Provot J, Jais JP, et al, Members of the CEREDIH French PID Study Group. Autoimmune and inflammatory manifestations occur frequently in patients with primary immunodeficiencies. J Allergy Clin Immunol 2017;140(5): 1388–93.e8.
62. Bacchetta R, Notarangelo LD. Immunodeficiency with autoimmunity: beyond the paradox. Front Immunol 2013;4:77.
63. Halfvarson J, Brislawn CJ, Lamendella R, et al. Dynamics of the human gut microbiome in inflammatory bowel disease. Nat Microbiol 2017;2:17004.
64. Gupta N, Bostrom AG, Kirschner BS, et al. Presentation and disease course in early- compared to later-onset pediatric Crohn's disease. Am J Gastroenterol 2008;103(8):2092–8.
65. Benchimol EI, Mack DR, Nguyen GC, et al. Incidence, outcomes, and health services burden of very early onset inflammatory bowel disease. Gastroenterology 2014;147(4):803–13.e7 [quiz: e814–5].
66. Oliva-Hemker M, Hutfless S, Al Kazzi ES, et al. Clinical presentation and five-year therapeutic management of very early-onset inflammatory bowel disease in a large North American cohort. J Pediatr 2015;167(3):527–32.e1-3.
67. Glocker EO, Kotlarz D, Boztug K, et al. Inflammatory bowel disease and mutations affecting the interleukin-10 receptor. N Engl J Med 2009;361(21):2033–45.
68. Uhlig HH, Schwerd T, Koletzko S, et al. The diagnostic approach to monogenic very early onset inflammatory bowel disease. Gastroenterology 2014;147(5): 990–1007.e3.

69. Ashton JJ, Harden A, Beattie RM. Paediatric inflammatory bowel disease: improving early diagnosis. Arch Dis Child 2018;103(4):307–8.

70. Meeths M, Entesarian M, Al-Herz W, et al. Spectrum of clinical presentations in familial hemophagocytic lymphohistiocytosis type 5 patients with mutations in STXBP2. Blood 2010;116(15):2635–43.

71. Levine AP, Pontikos N, Schiff ER, et al. Genetic complexity of Crohn's disease in two large Ashkenazi Jewish families. Gastroenterology 2016;151(4):698–709.

72. Speckmann C, Doerken S, Aiuti A, et al. A prospective study on the natural history of patients with profound combined immunodeficiency: an interim analysis. J Allergy Clin Immunol 2017;139(4):1302–10.e4.

73. Schwerd T, Bryant RV, Pandey S, et al. NOX1 loss-of-function genetic variants in patients with inflammatory bowel disease. Mucosal Immunol 2017;11:562–74.

74. Uzel G, Orange JS, Poliak N, et al. Complications of tumor necrosis factor-alpha blockade in chronic granulomatous disease-related colitis. Clin Infect Dis 2010; 51(12):1429–34.

Gastrointestinal Manifestations and Complications of Primary Immunodeficiency Disorders

Shradha Agarwal, MD*, Charlotte Cunningham-Rundles, MD, PhD

KEYWORDS

- Primary immunodeficiency disorder • Gastrointestinal tract
- Inflammatory bowel disease • Intestinal disease • Chronic enteropathy • Diarrhea

KEY POINTS

- The gastrointestinal tract mucosa is the largest immune system organ containing the majority of lymphocytes and immunoglobulins synthesized in the body.
- There is a wide range of infectious and noninfectious GI disease associated with primary immunodeficiency that can be the presenting symptom of immunodeficiency.
- Although symptoms of GI disease in immunodeficiency patients mimic those in immunocompetent patients, the pathologic factors and mechanism of disease are unique.
- Failure of GI diseases to respond to conventional treatment should prompt an evaluation for possible immunodeficiency.
- Further cellular and molecular understanding of the cause of GI involvement may provide more specific therapeutic options.

INTRODUCTION

Primary immunodeficiency disorders (PIDs) comprise more than 300 diseases characterized by defects across humoral, cellular, and phagocytic immunity.[1,2] Most PIDs share an increased susceptibility to infection, autoimmunity, and organ-specific disease. The gut-associated lymphoid tissue is the largest lymphoid organ in the body, with varying mechanisms for immune regulation; thus, dysregulation of immunity can manifest in a wide array of gastrointestinal (GI) diseases. Because of the complex

Disclosure Statement: Funding for this study was provided by the National Institutes of Health grants, AI-061093, AI-086037, AI-48693, and David S. Gottesman Immunology Chair at the Icahn School of Medicine at Mount Sinai.
Division of Allergy and Clinical Immunology after the Icahn School of Medicine at Mount Sinai, Icahn School of Medicine at Mount Sinai, One Gustave L. Levy Place, Box 1089, New York, NY 10029, USA
* Corresponding author.
E-mail address: shradha.agarwal@mssm.edu

Immunol Allergy Clin N Am 39 (2019) 81–94
https://doi.org/10.1016/j.iac.2018.08.006
0889-8561/19/© 2018 Elsevier Inc. All rights reserved.
immunology.theclinics.com

relationship between antigen tolerance and active immunity, GI disease in PIDs is often intractable and associated with significant morbidity and mortality.

Depending on the nature of the immune defect, GI disease ranges from 5% to 50% in PIDs. Diarrhea and malabsorption are common across many PIDs; whereas enteropathy may be more specific to PIDs with defects in more than 1 component of the immune system. This review highlights GI manifestations of common PIDs, focusing on symptom recognition, appropriate diagnostic studies, and therapies.

Selective IgA Deficiency

The most common primary immunodeficiency is selective IgA deficiency (sIgAD), defined as the absence of IgA (IgA <7 mg/dL) with normal or elevated levels of other immunoglobulins.[2] The prevalence varies among ethnicities from 1:100 to 1:1000.[3] Though the exact pathogenesis is not well-defined, decreased IgA production results from defects regulating terminal maturation of B-cells into IgA-secreting plasma cells.[2] Most sIgAD patients are asymptomatic, however, some individuals, more commonly those with concomitant IgG2 subclass deficiency, develop recurrent upper respiratory infections, autoimmune disorders, and allergic diseases.[2] IgA deficiency is associated with various autoimmune and inflammatory disorders of the gut. A 10- to 20- fold increase risk for celiac in sIgAD has been reported. The link between these diseases may be genetic through shared HLA haplotypes.[4] The histopathology and symptoms of celiac disease includes crypt hyperplasia, increased numbers of intraepithelial lymphocytes, villous flattening or shortening, and infiltration of the lamina propria with lymphoid cells resulting in malabsorption, diarrhea, steatorrhea, and weight loss. The absence of IgA-secreting plasma cells in intestinal biopsy specimens is characteristic of sIgAD. Thus, traditional screening tests using antiendomysial-IgA, antigliadin-IgA, and anti–tissue transglutaminase (tTG)-IgA antibodies are not reliable for diagnosis. Instead, IgG to deamidated gliadin peptides and tTG-IgG has been reported to be highly specific for diagnosing celiac disease in sIgAD.[4,5] Treatment includes elimination of gluten-containing foods, resulting in resolution of mucosal lesions and symptoms within a few weeks to months.[6]

Infections causing chronic diarrhea, commonly related to *Giardia lamblia*, occur with increased frequency[4] because lack of secretory IgA in sIgAD allows for attachment and proliferation of organisms on the intestinal epithelium.[7] *G lamblia* cysts give rise to trophozoites that colonize the small intestine and trigger bloating, cramping, excessive flatus, and watery diarrhea. Chronic infection can lead to steatorrhea and villus-flattening, and disruption of the absorption of lipids and carbohydrates. The degree of mucosal damage is associated with chronicity of infection and can cause irreversible epithelial damage. Diagnosis is made by examination of the stool for cysts or trophozoites of *G lamblia*, though duodenal aspirates may be more conclusive. Giardiasis is treated with amebicides; however, the parasitic burden can be unrelenting, requiring longer courses and/or alternative antimicrobials with more adverse profiles.

Nodular lymphoid hyperplasia (NLH) is characterized by numerous small nodules (usually 5 mm or larger) diffusely distributed along the GI tract in the lamina propria, superficial submucosa of the small intestine, or both. It is occasionally found in the stomach, large intestine, or rectum. NLH tends to have a benign course and usually regresses spontaneously in children. However, in adults, it is often associated with immunodeficiency with unclear prognosis.[8] Lesions can be associated with mucosal flattening, causing malabsorption, intussusception, and obstruction. Many patients are asymptomatic but may develop abdominal pain, chronic diarrhea, and bleeding. Diagnosis is made via endoscopy or barium study and confirmed by histologic findings, including hyperplastic, mitotically active germinal centers with well-defined lymphocyte mantles and lymphoid follicles. Immunohistochemical staining of sIgAD-associated NLH demonstrates large numbers of IgM-bearing cells, suggesting compensation for absent IgA.[9] Although there is no specific treatment, when discovered in the setting of G lamblia or Helicobacter pylori, eradication of the infection leads to regression of lymphoid nodules. Persistent NLH necessitates small bowel endoscopy with biopsy because NLH has been linked to lymphomas, usually B-cell tumors,[10] and gastric carcinomas.[11]

Other GI manifestations reported in sIgAD include chronic hepatitis, biliary cirrhosis, pernicious anemia, Crohn disease, and ulcerative colitis, although the prevalence of each is not well-defined.[4]

X-Linked Agammaglobulinemia

X-linked agammaglobulinemia (XLA), occurring in approximately 1 in 379,000 live births,[12] is an intrinsic B-cell disorder resulting from a defect in Bruton tyrosine kinase, causing arrest of pre-B cells and failure to generate mature B-cells. Peripheral CD19+ B cells are typically less than 2%, leading to a profound reduction in all immunoglobulin classes and depressed or absent humoral responses to specific antigens.[2]

GI manifestations are less common in XLA than other antibody deficiencies; however, in recent registry surveys, GI manifestations were reported in 35% of XLA patients.[13] Inflammatory bowel disease or enteritis in up to 10%, suggesting an effect of B cells on regulatory T cells (Tregs).[14] Chronic diarrhea that causes malabsorption is the most common manifestation, along with infectious diarrhea from G lamblia, Salmonella, Campylobacter, Cryptosporidium, and rotavirus.[15–17] Enteroviral infections, namely coxsackievirus and echovirus, can also cause meningoencephalitis.[18] Diagnosis can be made by cultures and/or polymerase chain reaction (PCR) assays. GI infections are treated based on cultures or PCR, and may require longer treatment courses and parenteral nutrition. Rare cases of gastric adenocarcinoma and colorectal cancer have been described.[19,20]

Hyper-IgM Syndromes

Hyper-IgM (HIGM) syndromes are a group of disorders leading to loss of T-cell–driven immunoglobulin class-switch recombination and/or defective somatic hypermutation with impaired T-cell activation.[2,21] The most common cause are mutations in the gene-encoding CD40 ligand (CD40L), leading to X-linked disease; less frequent are autosomal recessive mutations in CD40, activation-induced cytidine deaminase, and uracil-DNA glycosylase. An autosomal dominant gain of function mutation in phosphoinositide 3-kinase catalytic delta component[22] and mutations in the IKBKG gene nuclear factor-kappa beta (NF-κβ) essential modulator (NEMO),[23] both of which demonstrate elevated serum IgM levels, have also been identified. The estimated frequency of CD40L deficiency is 2 per 1,000,000 male patients, and autosomal mutations are even rarer.[24] T-lymphocyte numbers are typically normal and B-cell numbers are normal or slightly reduced. Patients have significantly low or absent levels of IgG and IgA, and normal or elevated levels of IgM. IgG response to vaccinations is poor or nonprotective. Patients with HIGM present early in life with recurrent sinopulmonary bacterial infections due to Streptococcus pneumoniae and Pseudomonas aeruginosa; however, opportunistic infections are more likely to occur with X-linked HIGM and CD40 defects due to impairment in macrophage and T-cell activation.[25]

Infectious diarrhea and noninfectious diarrhea are the most frequent GI diseases reported.[24,26] Infectious diarrhea has been associated with Cryptosporidium, Giardia, Salmonella, or Entamoeba infection.[26,27] CD40L defects are suspected to increase risk of chronic Cryptosporidium infection and hepatic complications, including sclerosing cholangitis, cirrhosis, and cholangiocarcinoma requiring liver transplantation.[21,28,29] Boiling or filtering drinking water can reduce the risk of *Cryptosporidium* infection. One HIGM cohort study found that liver disease with persistent infection at diagnosis was a statistically significant predictor of mortality for patients treated with hematopoietic stem cell transplantation (HSCT).[30]

Aphthous ulcers, gingivitis, and rectal ulcers can be associated with chronic or intermittent neutropenia.[21] Malignancies of the liver and GI tract, including biliary duct, hepatocellular carcinomas, carcinoid of the pancreas, glucagonoma of the pancreas, and adenocarcinomas of the liver and gall bladder, have been reported in HIGM.[24,31]

Common Variable Immunodeficiency

Common variable immunodeficiency (CVID), a heterogeneous PID characterized by the loss of B-cell function, has an estimated prevalence of 1 in 25,000 to 50,000 in whites.[1,32] The pathogenesis for CVID has not been clearly delineated; however, mutations in an increasing number of genes associated with B-cell development, including BAFF, TACI, ICOS, CD20, CD19, CD81, and CD21, as well as, more recently, NFKB1, CTLA4, LRBA, PI3KCD, STAT3, and IKAROS have been identified.[1,32] In CVID there are significantly low levels of IgG associated with low IgA and/or IgM, and poor or absent specific antibody responses, with the exclusion of other genetic or medical causes of hypogammaglobinemia. Decreased numbers of isotype-switched memory B-cells (CD27+IgD-IgM-), increased numbers of CD21low B cells, and loss of plasma cells in bone marrow and tissue are characteristic. T-cell defects, including excess numbers of memory T cells, loss of T-cell proliferation, and T-cell–associated cytokine defects, can contribute to clinical phenotypes. Patients typically present with recurrent bacterial infections of the respiratory tract, autoimmune disease, granulomatous or lymphoid infiltrative disease, and increased incidence of malignancy.[33] Most patients are diagnosed between the ages of 20 and 40 years, although the diagnosis of CVID may be delayed by 6 to 8 years even after the onset of characteristic symptoms.

Various reviews have noted a higher incidence of both infectious and noninfectious GI diseases in CVID as compared with other antibody deficiencies, perhaps due to more global impairments in cellular function.[33–36]

Acute or chronic infectious diarrhea is the most common GI symptom associated with CVID (20%–60%), leading to weight loss and malnutrition. Prolonged courses of treatment for eradication may be required.[36,37] Newly available PCR testing can rapidly detect many bacteria, viruses, and parasites. *G lamblia* is the most common organism; however, *Campylobacter jejuni*, *Salmonella* spp, cytomegalovirus, and (more recently) norovirus have been reported.[16,35,38,39] Giardiasis can cause villous blunting, increased intraepithelial lymphocytes, and NLH. Despite the frequent use of antibiotics in CVID, there does not seem to be a higher incidence of *Clostridium difficile* infection, possibly due to high titers of anti–*C difficile* antibodies in immunoglobulin preparations that may leak into the gut.[40] In contrast, small intestine bacterial overgrowth is common. Diagnosis may be challenging due to intermittent or chronic antibiotic exposure; it requires a hydrogen breath test.

The *H pylori* infection rate in CVID is equivalent to the general population; however, has been associated with gastritis, gastric dysplasia, and gastric cancer in CVID.[41] Previous studies reported a 10-fold increased risk of gastric cancer in CVID compared with the general population; however, recent studies suggest the risk maybe lower.[33,41,42] In 1 cohort; 6 of 8 CVID subjects with *H pylori* infection had gastric intestinal metaplasia and pathologic factors that did not resolve with treatment.[38] Therefore, patients who do not respond clinically to treatment should have regular endoscopic surveillance. In another study, CVID-associated adenocarcinomas were found to be diagnosed at a younger age, were of intestinal type, and associated with increased numbers of intratumoral lymphocytes.[43]

Small bowel villous atrophy is frequent in CVID patients and is frequently associated with severe malabsorption, as well as bloating, diarrhea, and weight loss. Histopathology demonstrates short villi, crypt hyperplasia, intraepithelial lymphocytosis, and (in some cases), an increase in apoptotic bodies in crypt epithelial cells.[35,38,44] Plasma cells in the lamina propria are absent or reduced and patients do not produce antibodies to tTG, endomysium, or gliadin. Most patients do not respond to a gluten-free diet or bear the HLA genes associated with celiac disease, suggesting alternative dysregulation in disease pathogenesis.[38,45] Inflammation and symptoms respond to corticosteroid therapy, and immunomodulators such as 6-mercaptopurine (6MP) or azathioprine (AZA) can be used. In cases of severe malabsorption, significant loss of the essential nutrients calcium and zinc, and vitamins A, D, and E, may lead to bone loss and neurologic deficits. Limited use of total parenteral nutrition may be required, with risk of central venous catheter-related infections.

Approximately 10% of CVID patients present with evidence of liver damage, including chronic hepatitis, autoimmune hepatitis, primary biliary cirrhosis, primary sclerosing cholangitis, and cirrhosis, most commonly due to nodular regenerative hyperplasia, which can lead to chronic cholestasis and portal hypertension that is difficult to manage.[32,33,46,47] These patients may be asymptomatic or have fatigue, nausea, vomiting, jaundice, ascites, hepatosplenomegaly, and esophageal varices.[46,48] Laboratory tests, and other liver function tests, show elevated alkaline phosphatase, with or without significant increases in bilirubin. In CVID, imaging to evaluate structural changes and liver biopsy are required for diagnosis. Biopsy demonstrates nonspecific portal and lobular inflammation, interface hepatitis, lymphocyte infiltration without plasma cells, granulomas, fibrosis, macrovesicular steatosis, and neogenesis of biliary ducts.[47,48] Current therapies for autoimmune liver disease in CVID include corticosteroids or immunomodulators[49–51]; ursodeoxycholic acid can be used if biliary damage is evident.[52] Liver transplant for cirrhosis has been reported[53]; however, a recent study demonstrated a statistically significant decrease in survival after liver transplantation for CVID-related liver disease (55% at 3 and 5 years).[54]

Malignancies are more frequent in patients with CVID compared with the general population, with lymphomas most commonly reported.[32,33,42] Non-Hodgkin B-cell lymphomas, Epstein-Barr virus–negative, predominate and often involve extra nodal sites, including the GI tract. CVID patients may develop NLH distributed diffusely throughout the stomach, ileum, and colon, which can result in intestinal obstruction and intussusception, as well as malabsorption. Immunohistochemical and gene rearrangement studies can be helpful in evaluating cases of atypical lymphoid hyperplasia; however, identification of clonal B-cell expansion may not be diagnostic.[55] Treatment of CVID-associated lymphoma is similar to that of other lymphomas and may include rituximab with cyclophosphamide, doxorubicin, vincristine, and prednisone (CHOP).

Approximately 10% to 20% of patients develop granulomatous disease. Most are noncaseating granulomas found in the lung, lymph node, or liver; however, they have also been reported in the GI tract, causing diarrhea and weight loss. Granulomatous disease in CVID is difficult to treat but biological therapies such as infliximab and rituximab have been used.[49]

Inflammatory bowel disease (IBD) resembling Crohn or ulcerative colitis has been reported in CVID cohorts[33–35,44,56] with weight loss, chronic diarrhea, rectal bleeding, abdominal pain, and malabsorption. IBD-like disease is typically diagnosed after the diagnosis of CVID but can be the presenting condition. Endoscopic features include longitudinal ulcers and cobblestone appearance. Histologically, it can mimic lymphocytic colitis, collagenous colitis, and colitis associated with graft-versus-host disease.[44,57] Tissue pathologic assessment reveals increased numbers of CD8+ T-cell infiltrates in the lamina propria, with a paucity of plasma cells. Furthermore, lamina propria mononuclear cells of CVID patients may produce more interleukin (IL)-12 and interferon-γ but not IL-23 and IL-17 compared with controls, suggesting an alternative pathway of inflammation.[56]

Immunoglobulin replacement does not ameliorate IBD-like disease, and use of corticosteroids increases infectious susceptibility. Treatment of CVID-associated colitis includes antibiotics to eliminate bacterial overgrowth, oral budesonide, 5-aminosalicylate agents, 6MP, and AZA.[58] These medications do not significantly compromise immune function and immunoglobulin replacement helps protect patients from infectious complications to some degree. Gut inflammation in CVID is often difficult to control and unresponsive to standard IBD therapies. Targeted biological therapies, such as infliximab, adalimumab, and ustekinumab, have been used with some benefit in cases of severe enteropathy; however, patients with significant T-cell defects require monitoring for fungal infections,[59–61] and the duration of treatment is not established. There is some concern that the use of the anti-$\alpha4\beta7$ integrin vedolizumab could potentially worsen enteropathy by blocking extravasation of Tregs into the gut mucosa[60] but this therapy has been used with some success.[62]

Chronic Granulomatous Disease

Chronic granulomatous disease (CGD), affecting 1 in 200,000 US births, is caused by the inability of phagocytes to produce adequate reactive oxygen metabolites to kill ingested microorganisms owing to abnormalities in components of nicotinamide adenine dinucleotide phosphate (NADPH) oxidase, with the most common form being X-linked (gp91^{phox}) and others being autosomal recessive.[2] Most individuals present with recurrent infections by catalase-positive organisms, such as *Staphylococcus aureus*, *Burkholderia cepacia*, *Serratia marcescens*, *Aspergillus* sp, *Chromobacterium violaceu*, *and Nocardia* sp, at epithelial surfaces (skin, gut, lungs), as well as in organs with a large numbers of reticuloendothelial cells, such as the liver.[63] Diagnosis is established by flow cytometry demonstrating defective oxidation of dihydrorhodamine by neutrophils and genetics to confirm the inheritance pattern.[2]

GI involvement occurs in approximately 80% of patients with CGD, ranging from noninfectious diarrhea, oral aphthae, anal fistula, and abdominal pain. The rate of gut involvement has been reported to be higher in X-linked gp91^{phox} deficiency compared with autosomal recessive forms. Intestinal dysmotility, obstruction, and ulcerations can occur along the entire length of the GI tract, with the colon being most frequently involved.[63] The presence of perianal disease and rectal abscesses in infancy are clinically suggestive of CGD. Granulomas, giant cells, and macrophages laden with brown-yellow fine pigment are present in gastric biopsies. It is speculated that chronic antigenic stimulation from organisms persisting within phagocytes results in granuloma formation and bowel wall thickening.[64] These may resolve after treatment with corticosteroids and antibiotics but in many cases require surgery.

An IBD phenotype with gut inflammation is frequently chronic and relapsing.[64] Patients present with recurrent diarrhea, anal fissures, perirectal abscesses, and GI tract obstruction.[65] Endoscopy can reveal colonic narrowing, cobblestone pattern, thickened bowel wall, fistulization, pancolitis, patchy friability, pseudopolyps, and/or hemorrhage.[65,66] Inflammation is typically discontinuous and the perianal area is frequently involved. Histopathologic findings include acute and chronic inflammatory infiltrates, granulomas (usually in the muscularis), submucosal edema, and crypt abscesses. CGD-unique elements include lack of neutrophils, increased eosinophils, eosinophilic cryptitis, and pigment-laden macrophages in the lamina propria.[66,67] A high rate of antimicrobial antibodies are present in CGD-associated colitis, with 1 study sequencing Acetobacteraceae from patient granulomas.[68]

Treatment is not well-defined; however, infectious causes should be excluded and treated with agents targeting bacterial and fungal pathogens. Systemic steroids or ileal-release budesonide has been initiated after biopsy confirmation of granuloma but relapses are common on discontinuation.[66,69] Steroid-sparing agents, including 5-aminosalicylates, thiopurines, methotrexate, cyclosporine, and antitumor necrosis factor-α, are other options, though reports of infectious complications may preclude their use in CGD.[66,70] Treatment with granulocyte-macrophage colony-stimulating factor and granulocyte colony-stimulating factor have also been investigated.[71,72] Surgery may be considered in patients with refractory colitis. Bone marrow transplantation can be offered to those with complicated disease and a suitable stem cell match.[73]

Liver involvement in CGD is common, frequently as abscesses; however, nodular regenerative hyperplasia, portal hypertension, and hepatosplenomegaly also occur. Hepatic abscesses, reported in up to 32% of patients, may be recurrent, numerous, and prolonged.[69,74] Patients may present with elevated transaminases, fever, abdominal pain, weight loss, and night sweats. *Staphylococcus aureus* is the most common organism identified in liver abscesses. A low threshold for imaging is required for diagnosis. Treatment requires extensive surgical drainage and debridement with appropriate antimicrobial agents. More recently, the combination of extensive antibiotic therapy with prolonged corticosteroids has been used with success, demonstrating the excessive inflammatory nature of these lesions.[74] A small portion of CGD patients develop progressive noncirrhotic portal hypertension due to microvasculature damage from repeated liver abscesses. Diminishing platelet counts may be used as a clinical indicator of disease progression.

Severe Combined Immunodeficiency

Severe combined immunodeficiency (SCID) is a group of congenital disorders characterized by severe impairment in T-cell, B-cell, and natural killer (NK) cell function. It is classified as T-B + NK+, T-B + NK-, T-B-NK+, or T-B-NK- based on the presence or absence of defects affecting these cells. Several molecular defects, including but not limited to mutations in adenosine deaminase, purine nucleoside phosphorylase, Zeta-chain-associated protein kinase 70 (ZAP 70), Janus kinase 3 (JAK3), recombination-activating genes (RAG 1/2), IL-7 receptor- α, and IL2-Rγ chain have been reported to result in the SCID phenotype.[1] SCID prevalence is estimated at 1 in 50,000 live births, but may be more frequent in cultures with consanguineous marriages. The diagnosis is suspected when the absolute lymphocyte count is less than 2500 cells/mm,[3] CD3+ T cells are less than 20%, and proliferative responses to mitogens are less than 10% of the control. Serum levels of immunoglobulins are usually very low and specific antibody responses are impaired. In the absence of bone marrow transplantation, SCID is fatal. Newborn screening using dried blood spots to measure T-cell receptor excision circles has been instituted in almost all states, leading to early recognition of these infants.[2]

Before newborn screening, infants with SCID presented in the first year of life with severe bacterial, viral, and opportunistic infections, usually of the lung and GI tract; eczematous rashes; and failure to thrive. Oral, esophageal, and perianal candidiasis is common, often affecting nutritional status. Affected children develop severe, chronic diarrhea, malabsorption, and growth impairment early in life. Cultures for bacterial, fungal, and viral pathogens are essential, and identification may require PCR and histopathological examination of the tissue. GI infections with cytomegalovirus and rotavirus are common and may cause persistent diarrhea and malabsorption.

Picornavirus, parvovirus, adenovirus, *Salmonella*, *G lamblia*, *Escherichia coli*, and *Cryptosporidium* have also been isolated.[75] Intestinal biopsies demonstrate hypocellular lamina propria without plasma cells or lymphocytes and villous atrophy occurs in some infants owing to infection-related intestinal damage.[44] SCID patients receiving blood transfusions or allogenic bone marrow transplant are susceptible to graft-versus-host disease, which may affect the colon and small intestine.

Immune Dysfunction, Polyendocrinopathy, Enteropathy, X-Linked Syndrome

Immune dysfunction, polyendocrinopathy, enteropathy, X-linked (IPEX) syndrome is due to the loss of function mutations in the FOXP3 gene, a transcriptional regulator required for Tregs and maintenance of peripheral tolerance.[76,77] The exact prevalence is unknown. IPEX patients present within the first few months of life with multiple autoimmune manifestations, diabetes mellitus, eczematous dermatitis, thyroiditis, thrombocytopenia, and severe enteropathy.[78] Serum IgG, IgA, and IgM levels are usually normal; however, IgG can be reduced from enteric protein loss. Total and antigen-specific IgE are usually elevated and eosinophilia may also be present. Affected patients typically have decreased numbers of Tregs and are unable to suppress T-cell proliferation.[79] Diagnosis is made by demonstrating decreased FOXP3 protein expression and reduced numbers of Tregs; definitive diagnosis requires gene sequencing to identify FOXP3 gene mutations.[80]

The most consistent feature of IPEX is chronic intractable diarrhea, usually watery but also mucoid or bloody, with failure to thrive due to enteropathy and malabsorption.[81] Histopathologic findings include destruction of small bowel mucosa due to total or partial villous atrophy, ulcerations, and hyperemic mucosa. Involvement of the large intestine can occur with lymphocytic and plasma cell infiltrates in the lamina propria and presence of eosinophils.

Patients are often severely ill due to malnutrition, electrolyte imbalance, or infection by the time IPEX is diagnosed. In the absence of aggressive therapy and HSCT, IPEX can be fatal before 2 years of age.[82] HSCT has resulted in gut immune reconstitution and improved colitis.[83,84] Symptomatic treatment of GI disease includes bowel rest with total parenteral nutrition. Immunosuppressive agents, such as cyclosporine A, tacrolimus (FK506), sirolimus, and corticosteroids have been used with some success; however, long-term treatment may be challenging due to toxicity and underlying immune suppression,[85–87] and may facilitate opportunistic infections.[88,89]

SUMMARY

Although the hallmark of PIDs is increased susceptibility to infection, many are associated with and initially present with GI diseases, making routine evaluation of the gut necessary. A history of recurrent infections, clinical and/or histologic features atypical of the usual pattern of GI disease, or a poor response to conventional therapy should prompt further immunologic evaluation. Early diagnosis and treatment may prevent irreversible tissue damage and mortality. In most cases, treatment with replacement immunoglobulin and antibiotics does not reverse or prevent the development of GI disease; therefore, additional immunomodulatory therapies, including, in some cases, organ transplantation, are indicated.

REFERENCES

1. Picard C, Bobby Gaspar H, Al-Herz W, et al. International Union of Immunological Societies: 2017 primary immunodeficiency diseases committee report on inborn errors of immunity. J Clin Immunol 2018;38(1):96–128.

2. Bonilla FA, Khan DA, Ballas ZK, et al. Practice parameter for the diagnosis and management of primary immunodeficiency. J Allergy Clin Immunol 2015;136(5): 1186–205.e1-8.

3. Aghamohammadi A, Mohammadinejad P, Abolhassani H, et al. Primary immunodeficiency disorders in Iran: update and new insights from the third report of the national registry. J Clin Immunol 2014;34(4):478–90.

4. Yazdani R, Azizi G, Abolhassani H, et al. Selective IgA deficiency: epidemiology, pathogenesis, clinical phenotype, diagnosis, prognosis and management. Scand J Immunol 2017;85(1):3–12.

5. Villalta D, Alessio MG, Tampoia M, et al. Diagnostic accuracy of IgA anti-tissue transglutaminase antibody assays in celiac disease patients with selective IgA deficiency. Ann N Y Acad Sci 2007;1109:212–20.

6. Chow MA, Lebwohl B, Reilly NR, et al. Immunoglobulin A deficiency in celiac disease. J Clin Gastroenterol 2012;46(10):850–4.

7. Heyworth MF, Carlson JR, Ermak TH. Clearance of *Giardia muris* infection requires helper/inducer T lymphocytes. J Exp Med 1987;165(6):1743–8.

8. Basyigit S, Aktas B, Simsek H, et al. Diffuse intestinal nodular lymphoid hyperplasia in an immunoglobulin-A-deficient patient with *Helicobacter pylori* infection. Endoscopy 2014;46(Suppl 1 UCTN):E568–9.

9. Jacobson KW, deShazo RD. Selective immunoglobulin A deficiency associated with modular lymphoid hyperplasia. J Allergy Clin Immunol 1979;64(6 Pt 1): 516–21.

10. Hanich T, Majnaric L, Jankovic D, et al. Nodular lymphoid hyperplasia complicated with ileal Burkitt's lymphoma in an adult patient with selective IgA deficiency. Int J Surg Case Rep 2017;30:69–72.

11. Mir-Madjlessi SH, Vafai M, Khademi J, et al. Coexisting primary malignant lymphoma and adenocarcinoma of the large intestine in an IgA-deficient boy. Dis Colon Rectum 1984;27(12):822–4.

12. Winkelstein JA, Marino MC, Lederman HM, et al. X-linked agammaglobulinemia: report on a United States registry of 201 patients. Medicine (Baltimore) 2006; 85(4):193–202.

13. Barmettler S, Otani IM, Minhas J, et al. Gastrointestinal manifestations in X-linked agammaglobulinemia. J Clin Immunol 2017;37(3):287–94.

14. Hernandez-Trujillo VP, Scalchunes C, Cunningham-Rundles C, et al. Autoimmunity and inflammation in X-linked agammaglobulinemia. J Clin Immunol 2014; 34(6):627–32.

15. Atarod L, Raissi A, Aghamohammadi A, et al. A review of gastrointestinal disorders in patients with primary antibody immunodeficiencies during a 10-year period (1990-2000), in children hospital medical center. Iran J Allergy Asthma Immunol 2003;2(2):75–9.

16. van de Ven AA, Janssen WJ, Schulz LS, et al. Increased prevalence of gastrointestinal viruses and diminished secretory immunoglobulin a levels in antibody deficiencies. J Clin Immunol 2014;34(8):962–70.

17. Pac M, Bernatowska EA, Kierkus J, et al. Gastrointestinal disorders next to respiratory infections as leading symptoms of X-linked agammaglobulinemia in children - 34-year experience of a single center. Arch Med Sci 2017;13(2):412–7.

18. Quartier P, Foray S, Casanova JL, et al. Enteroviral meningoencephalitis in X-linked agammaglobulinemia: intensive immunoglobulin therapy and sequential viral detection in cerebrospinal fluid by polymerase chain reaction. Pediatr Infect Dis J 2000;19(11):1106–8.

19. van der Meer JW, Weening RS, Schellekens PT, et al. Colorectal cancer in patients with X-linked agammaglobulinaemia. Lancet 1993;341(8858):1439–40.
20. Staines Boone AT, Torres Martinez MG, Lopez Herrera G, et al. Gastric adenocarcinoma in the context of X-linked agammaglobulinemia: case report and review of the literature. J Clin Immunol 2014;34(2):134–7.
21. Davies EG, Thrasher AJ. Update on the hyper immunoglobulin M syndromes. Br J Haematol 2010;149(2):167–80.
22. Lucas CL, Kuehn HS, Zhao F, et al. Dominant-activating germline mutations in the gene encoding the PI(3)K catalytic subunit p110delta result in T cell senescence and human immunodeficiency. Nat Immunol 2014;15(1):88–97.
23. Zonana J, Elder ME, Schneider LC, et al. A novel X-linked disorder of immune deficiency and hypohidrotic ectodermal dysplasia is allelic to incontinentia pigmenti and due to mutations in IKK-gamma (NEMO). Am J Hum Genet 2000; 67(6):1555–62.
24. Winkelstein JA, Marino MC, Ochs H, et al. The X-linked hyper-IgM syndrome: clinical and immunologic features of 79 patients. Medicine (Baltimore) 2003;82(6): 373–84.
25. Fuleihan R, Ramesh N, Loh R, et al. Defective expression of the CD40 ligand in X chromosome-linked immunoglobulin deficiency with normal or elevated IgM. Proc Natl Acad Sci U S A 1993;90(6):2170–3.
26. Leven EA, Maffucci P, Ochs HD, et al. Hyper IgM syndrome: a report from the USIDNET registry. J Clin Immunol 2016;36(5):490–501.
27. Quartier P, Bustamante J, Sanal O, et al. Clinical, immunologic and genetic analysis of 29 patients with autosomal recessive hyper-IgM syndrome due to activation-induced cytidine deaminase deficiency. Clin Immunol 2004;110(1):22–9.
28. Dimicoli S, Bensoussan D, Latger-Cannard V, et al. Complete recovery from *Cryptosporidium parvum* infection with gastroenteritis and sclerosing cholangitis after successful bone marrow transplantation in two brothers with X-linked hyper-IgM syndrome. Bone Marrow Transplant 2003;32(7):733–7.
29. Azzu V, Kennard L, Morillo-Gutierrez B, et al. Liver disease predicts mortality in patients with X-linked immunodeficiency with hyper-IgM but can be prevented by early hematopoietic stem cell transplantation. J Allergy Clin Immunol 2018; 141(1):405–8.e7.
30. de la Morena MT, Leonard D, Torgerson TR, et al. Long-term outcomes of 176 patients with X-linked hyper-IgM syndrome treated with or without hematopoietic cell transplantation. J Allergy Clin Immunol 2017;139(4):1282–92.
31. Hayward AR, Levy J, Facchetti F, et al. Cholangiopathy and tumors of the pancreas, liver, and biliary tree in boys with X-linked immunodeficiency with hyper-IgM. J Immunol 1997;158(2):977–83.
32. Bonilla FA, Barlan I, Chapel H, et al. International Consensus Document (ICON): common variable immunodeficiency disorders. J Allergy Clin Immunol Pract 2016;4(1):38–59.
33. Resnick ES, Moshier EL, Godbold JH, et al. Morbidity and mortality in common variable immune deficiency over 4 decades. Blood 2012;119(7):1650–7.
34. Agarwal S, Smereka P, Harpaz N, et al. Characterization of immunologic defects in patients with common variable immunodeficiency (CVID) with intestinal disease. Inflamm Bowel Dis 2011;17(1):251–9.
35. Daniels JA, Lederman HM, Maitra A, et al. Gastrointestinal tract pathology in patients with common variable immunodeficiency (CVID): a clinicopathologic study and review. Am J Surg Pathol 2007;31(12):1800–12.

36. Oksenhendler E, Gerard L, Fieschi C, et al. Infections in 252 patients with common variable immunodeficiency. Clin Infect Dis 2008;46(10):1547–54.
37. Pecoraro A, Nappi L, Crescenzi L, et al. Chronic diarrhea in common variable immunodeficiency: a case series and review of the literature. J Clin Immunol 2018; 38(1):67–76.
38. Malamut G, Verkarre V, Suarez F, et al. The enteropathy associated with common variable immunodeficiency: the delineated frontiers with celiac disease. Am J Gastroenterol 2010;105(10):2262–75.
39. Woodward JM, Gkrania-Klotsas E, Cordero-Ng AY, et al. The role of chronic norovirus infection in the enteropathy associated with common variable immunodeficiency. Am J Gastroenterol 2015;110(2):320–7.
40. Salcedo J, Keates S, Pothoulakis C, et al. Intravenous immunoglobulin therapy for severe *Clostridium difficile* colitis. Gut 1997;41(3):366–70.
41. Dhalla F, da Silva SP, Lucas M, et al. Review of gastric cancer risk factors in patients with common variable immunodeficiency disorders, resulting in a proposal for a surveillance programme. Clin Exp Immunol 2011;165(1):1–7.
42. Gathmann B, Mahlaoui N, CEREDIH, et al. Clinical picture and treatment of 2212 patients with common variable immunodeficiency. J Allergy Clin Immunol 2014; 134(1):116–26.
43. De Petris G, Dhungel BM, Chen L, et al. Gastric adenocarcinoma in common variable immunodeficiency: features of cancer and associated gastritis may be characteristic of the condition. Int J Surg Pathol 2014;22(7):600–6.
44. Washington K, Stenzel TT, Buckley RH, et al. Gastrointestinal pathology in patients with common variable immunodeficiency and X-linked agammaglobulinemia. Am J Surg Pathol 1996;20(10):1240–52.
45. Biagi F, Bianchi PI, Zilli A, et al. The significance of duodenal mucosal atrophy in patients with common variable immunodeficiency: a clinical and histopathologic study. Am J Clin Pathol 2012;138(2):185–9.
46. Ward C, Lucas M, Piris J, et al. Abnormal liver function in common variable immunodeficiency disorders due to nodular regenerative hyperplasia. Clin Exp Immunol 2008;153(3):331–7.
47. Daniels JA, Torbenson M, Vivekanandan P, et al. Hepatitis in common variable immunodeficiency. Hum Pathol 2009;40(4):484–8.
48. Fukushima K, Ueno Y, Kanegane H, et al. A case of severe recurrent hepatitis with common variable immunodeficiency. Hepatol Res 2008;38(4):415–20.
49. Boursiquot JN, Gerard L, Malphettes M, et al. Granulomatous disease in CVID: retrospective analysis of clinical characteristics and treatment efficacy in a cohort of 59 patients. J Clin Immunol 2013;33(1):84–95.
50. Thatayatikom A, Thatayatikom S, White AJ. Infliximab treatment for severe granulomatous disease in common variable immunodeficiency: a case report and review of the literature. Ann Allergy Asthma Immunol 2005;95(3):293–300.
51. Franxman TJ, Howe LE, Baker JR Jr. Infliximab for treatment of granulomatous disease in patients with common variable immunodeficiency. J Clin Immunol 2014;34(7):820–7.
52. Xiao X, Miao Q, Chang C, et al. Common variable immunodeficiency and autoimmunity–an inconvenient truth. Autoimmun Rev 2014;13(8):858–64.
53. Montalti R, Mocchegiani F, Vincenzi P, et al. Liver transplantation in patients with common variable immunodeficiency: a report of two cases. Ann Transplant 2014; 19:541–4.

54. Azzu V, Elias JE, Duckworth A, et al. Liver transplantation in adults with liver disease due to common variable immunodeficiency leads to early recurrent disease and poor outcome. Liver Tanspl 2018;24(2):171–81.

55. Sander CA, Medeiros LJ, Weiss LM, et al. Lymphoproliferative lesions in patients with common variable immunodeficiency syndrome. Am J Surg Pathol 1992; 16(12):1170–82.

56. Mannon PJ, Fuss IJ, Dill S, et al. Excess IL-12 but not IL-23 accompanies the inflammatory bowel disease associated with common variable immunodeficiency. Gastroenterology 2006;131(3):748–56.

57. Byrne MF, Royston D, Patchett SE. Association of common variable immunodeficiency with atypical collagenous colitis. Eur J Gastroenterol Hepatol 2003;15(9): 1051–3.

58. Elnachef N, McMorris M, Chey WD. Successful treatment of common variable immunodeficiency disorder-associated diarrhea with budesonide: a case report. Am J Gastroenterol 2007;102(6):1322–5.

59. Chua I, Standish R, Lear S, et al. Anti-tumour necrosis factor-alpha therapy for severe enteropathy in patients with common variable immunodeficiency (CVID). Clin Exp Immunol 2007;150(2):306–11.

60. Uzzan M, Ko HM, Mehandru S, et al. Gastrointestinal Disorders Associated with Common Variable Immune Deficiency (CVID) and Chronic Granulomatous Disease (CGD). Curr Gastroenterol Rep 2016;18(4):17.

61. Ruiz de Morales JG, Munoz F, Hernando M. Successful treatment of common variable immunodeficiency-associated inflammatory bowel disease with Ustekinumab. J Crohns Colitis 2017;11(9):1154–5.

62. Boland BS, Riedl MA, Valasek MA, et al. Vedolizumab in patients with common variable immune deficiency and gut inflammation. Am J Gastroenterol 2017; 112(10):1621.

63. Magnani A, Brosselin P, Beaute J, et al. Inflammatory manifestations in a single-center cohort of patients with chronic granulomatous disease. J Allergy Clin Immunol 2014;134(3):655–62.e8.

64. Yu JE, De Ravin SS, Uzel G, et al. High levels of Crohn's disease-associated antimicrobial antibodies are present and independent of colitis in chronic granulomatous disease. Clin Immunol 2011;138(1):14–22.

65. Huang A, Abbasakoor F, Vaizey CJ. Gastrointestinal manifestations of chronic granulomatous disease. Colorectal Dis 2006;8(8):637–44.

66. Marks DJ, Miyagi K, Rahman FZ, et al. Inflammatory bowel disease in CGD reproduces the clinicopathological features of Crohn's disease. Am J Gastroenterol 2009;104(1):117–24.

67. Alimchandani M, Lai JP, Aung PP, et al. Gastrointestinal histopathology in chronic granulomatous disease: a study of 87 patients. Am J Surg Pathol 2013;37(9): 1365–72.

68. Greenberg DE, Ding L, Zelazny AM, et al. A novel bacterium associated with lymphadenitis in a patient with chronic granulomatous disease. PLoS Pathog 2006;2(4):e28.

69. Marciano BE, Rosenzweig SD, Kleiner DE, et al. Gastrointestinal involvement in chronic granulomatous disease. Pediatrics 2004;114(2):462–8.

70. Rosh JR, Tang HB, Mayer L, et al. Treatment of intractable gastrointestinal manifestations of chronic granulomatous disease with cyclosporine. J Pediatr 1995; 126(1):143–5.

71. Wang J, Mayer L, Cunningham-Rundles C. Use of GM-CSF in the treatment of colitis associated with chronic granulomatous disease. J Allergy Clin Immunol 2005; 115(5):1092–4.

72. Myrup B, Valerius NH, Mortensen PB. Treatment of enteritis in chronic granulomatous disease with granulocyte colony stimulating factor. Gut 1998;42(1):127–30.

73. Gungor T, Teira P, Slatter M, et al. Reduced-intensity conditioning and HLA-matched haemopoietic stem-cell transplantation in patients with chronic granulomatous disease: a prospective multicentre study. Lancet 2014; 383(9915):436–48.

74. Leiding JW, Freeman AF, Marciano BE, et al. Corticosteroid therapy for liver abscess in chronic granulomatous disease. Clin Infect Dis 2012;54(5):694–700.

75. Stephan JL, Vlekova V, Le Deist F, et al. Severe combined immunodeficiency: a retrospective single-center study of clinical presentation and outcome in 117 patients. J Pediatr 1993;123(4):564–72.

76. Bennett CL, Christie J, Ramsdell F, et al. The immune dysregulation, polyendocrinopathy, enteropathy, X-linked syndrome (IPEX) is caused by mutations of FOXP3. Nat Genet 2001;27(1):20–1.

77. Bin Dhuban K, Piccirillo CA. The immunological and genetic basis of immune dysregulation, polyendocrinopathy, enteropathy, X-linked syndrome. Curr Opin Allergy Clin Immunol 2015;15(6):525–32.

78. Torgerson TR, Ochs HD. Immune dysregulation, polyendocrinopathy, enteropathy, X-linked: forkhead box protein 3 mutations and lack of regulatory T cells. J Allergy Clin Immunol 2007;120(4):744–50 [quiz: 751–2].

79. d'Hennezel E, Ben-Shoshan M, Ochs HD, et al. FOXP3 forkhead domain mutation and regulatory T cells in the IPEX syndrome. N Engl J Med 2009; 361(17):1710–3.

80. Seghezzo S, Bleesing JJ, Kucuk ZY. Persistent enteropathy in a toddler with a novel FOXP3 mutation and normal FOXP3 protein expression. J Pediatr 2017; 186:183–5.

81. Chandrakasan S, Venkateswaran S, Kugathasan S. Nonclassic inflammatory bowel disease in young infants: immune dysregulation, polyendocrinopathy, enteropathy, X-linked syndrome, and other disorders. Pediatr Clin North Am 2017; 64(1):139–60.

82. Kucuk ZY, Bleesing JJ, Marsh R, et al. A challenging undertaking: stem cell transplantation for immune dysregulation, polyendocrinopathy, enteropathy, X-linked (IPEX) syndrome. J Allergy Clin Immunol 2016;137(3):953–5.e4.

83. Rao A, Kamani N, Filipovich A, et al. Successful bone marrow transplantation for IPEX syndrome after reduced-intensity conditioning. Blood 2007;109(1):383–5.

84. Gambineri E, Ciullini Mannurita S, Robertson H, et al. Gut immune reconstitution in immune dysregulation, polyendocrinopathy, enteropathy, X-linked syndrome after hematopoietic stem cell transplantation. J Allergy Clin Immunol 2015; 135(1):260–2.

85. Kobayashi I, Kawamura N, Okano M. A long-term survivor with the immune dysregulation, polyendocrinopathy, enteropathy, X-linked syndrome. N Engl J Med 2001;345(13):999–1000.

86. Battaglia M, Stabilini A, Migliavacca B, et al. Rapamycin promotes expansion of functional CD4+CD25+FOXP3+ regulatory T cells of both healthy subjects and type 1 diabetic patients. J Immunol 2006;177(12):8338–47.

87. Yong PL, Russo P, Sullivan KE. Use of sirolimus in IPEX and IPEX-like children. J Clin Immunol 2008;28(5):581–7.

88. Lucas KG, Ungar D, Comito M, et al. Epstein Barr virus induced lymphoma in a child with IPEX syndrome. Pediatr Blood Cancer 2008;50(5):1056–7.
89. Taddio A, Faleschini E, Valencic E, et al. Medium-term survival without haematopoietic stem cell transplantation in a case of IPEX: insights into nutritional and immunosuppressive therapy. Eur J Pediatr 2007;166(11):1195–7.

Personalized Therapy
Immunoglobulin Replacement for Antibody Deficiency

Richard L. Wasserman, MD, PhD

KEYWORDS

- Antibody deficiency • IgG • Immunoglobulin • IVIG • SCIG • fSCIG

KEY POINTS

- Immunoglobulin G (IgG) replacement therapy is indicated for primary immunodeficiency disorder patients with a demonstrated antibody production defect.
- The ideal immunoglobulin (IG) dose for an individual patient is the dose that keeps the patient well.
- Personalization of IG therapy requires an understanding of the options for different modes of administration.
- Shared decision-making, engaging the patient and family in determining the mode of administration, enhances adherence.

INTRODUCTION

Passive immunization by administration of immunoglobulin G (IgG) from another organism originated with Behring's use of antitoxin to diphtheria and tetanus in the late 19th century. The identification of the first primary immunodeficiency disease (PIDD) patients was accompanied by the use of therapeutic human serum antibody in 1952.[1] Since 1952, immunoglobulin (IG) therapy has progressed to the point that there are several modalities available with which to treat patients. The introduction, in 1981, of an intravenous product[2] allowed a dramatic increase in dose that altered the outcome for many PIDD patients. The addition of commercial subcutaneous (2006)[3] and a facilitated subcutaneous product (2014)[4] provided important options for PIDD patients. Optimization of antibody deficiency patient outcomes requires an understanding of IG therapy and the modes of IG administration. A brief history of PIDD and IG therapy is shown in **Box 1**.

Disclosures: Investigator – CSL Behring, Korean Green Cross, Prometic, Shire, TherapureBio, Consultant – ADMA Biologics, Grifols, Korean Green Cross, Shire, TherapureBio. Speaker – Shire.
Allergy Partners of North Texas, 7777 Forest Lane, Suite B-332, Dallas, TX 75230, USA
E-mail address: drrichwasserman@gmail.com

Immunol Allergy Clin N Am 39 (2019) 95–111
https://doi.org/10.1016/j.iac.2018.08.001   immunology.theclinics.com
0889-8561/19/© 2018 Elsevier Inc. All rights reserved.

Box 1
History of primary immunodeficiency and immunoglobulin therapy

- Colonel Ogden Bruton 1952
  - Two brothers with recurrent pneumococcal bacteremia and absent gamma globulins
  - Treatment with subcutaneous gamma globulin prevented bacteremia
  - Addition of "spreading factor" enhanced subcutaneous infusions
  - Recurrent upper and lower respiratory tract infections continued

- 1950s to 1980s
  - Many immunodeficiency phenotypes reported
  - IG therapy went from SC to IM to IV

- 1990s
  - First immunodeficiency genotypes reported

- 2006
  - First SCIG product approved in the United States

- 2017
  - More than 350 immunodeficiency genotypes

Abbreviations: IG, immunoglobulin; IM, intramuscular; IV, intravenous, SC, subcutaneous.

Indications for Immunoglobulin Replacement

IG is used to provide passive immunity to patients with defective antibody production and is an immunomodulator. Although many PIDD patients have autoimmune diatheses, the focus of this article is the optimization of IG supplementation for PIDD patients with antibody production disorders. Therefore, the immunomodulatory uses of IG will not be discussed further except to note that because the dose, infusion frequencies, and outcome measures applied to IG therapy for immunomodulation are different than those used for the provision of passive immunity, not all of the recommendations in this article can be translated to other uses of IG.

The goal of replacement IG therapy is to prevent infection by passive immunization. Therefore, candidates for IG therapy must have a disorder of antibody production. This should be suggested by a history of recurrent infection, but the diagnosis of a classical immunodeficiency characterized by defective antibody production is made by either genetic or serum testing or appropriate laboratory evaluation to justify the administration of supplementary IgG. Although further studies may be useful to more fully characterize the phenotypic expression of the particular PIDD, therapy should not be delayed awaiting results. See **Box 2**

Box 2
Diagnostic criteria for IgG replacement in PIDD

Genetic diagnosis of PIDD mandating immediate IG treatment
- X-linked agammaglobulinemia
- Hyper IgM syndrome
- Severe combined immunodeficiency
- Wiskott-Aldrich syndrome

Recurrent bacterial infections AND

Evidence of an antibody production disorder
- Hypogammaglobulinemia
- Poor response to protein antigens—diphtheria and tetanus toxoid
- Poor response to carbohydrate antigens—pneumococcal polysaccharide vaccine

for a partial list of PIDDs that may be treated with IG replacement based on genetic diagnosis alone.

In 2018, recurrent infection is the more common presentation of immunodeficiency. Because IgG, in general, functions against prokaryotic organisms present in the interstitial space (as opposed to intracellular or eukaryotic pathogens), infections with common organisms, such as *Streptococcus pneumoniae*, *Haemophilus influenzae* and *Moraxella catarrhalis*, in common locations, such as sinuses, middle ear, and lungs, are the most common in patients with deficient antibody production although there may also be a history of cutaneous and gastroenterologic infections. Other susceptibility factors for infection, abnormalities at the intracellular (chronic granulomatous disease), organelle (cilia dysmotility syndrome, cystic fibrosis), or organ level (tracheo-esophageal fistula, recurrent aspiration), must be considered. In some patients an abnormal infection history is suggested by improper diagnosis (eg, viral upper respiratory tract infection or allergic rhinitis diagnosed as bacterial sinusitis or asthma diagnosed as recurrent pneumonia). For these reasons, a history of recurrent infection alone, without demonstrating defective antibody production, is insufficient justification for IG therapy.

In most patients, the minimal humoral immunity evaluation comprises measurement of concentrations of IgA, IgG, and IgM in blood and a demonstration of responsiveness to protein and polysaccharide antigens by the production of specific IgG antibody after antigen exposure. Although the determination of IG concentrations is straightforward, interpretation may be confounded by several factors. Normal IG concentrations vary by age until the late teenage years, so results must be interpreted in the context of the age-related normal values. In addition, there may be substantial variation between laboratories that should be considered when using information from serial measurements of IgG to influence the decision to treat with IG. The third, most difficult, issue relates to the predictive value of a particular IgG concentration, because there is not a close correlation between IgG concentration and infection susceptibility (see later discussion).

In addition to IG levels, the response to pneumococcal polysaccharide vaccine is used to assess the anticarbohydrate response and the diphtheria/tetanus vaccine response to assess the antiprotein response. Specific antibody responses to other antigens have been used. The use of vaccines in the diagnosis of PIDD and controversies regarding the interpretation of the results has been reviewed elsewhere.[5]

Although interpreting the data of a humoral immunodeficiency evaluation is straightforward for most patients, the results must be considered in the context of the patient's infection history, keeping in mind that the correlation between test results and infection susceptibility is imperfect. Because IG therapy is costly, clinicians should be mindful of insurance company laboratory diagnostic requirements to support the use of IG therapy.

History of Immunoglobulin Therapy

The use of blood proteins to provide passive immunity was first described in the late 19th century by Behring.[6] By the time Bruton identified the first PIDD patients in the early 1950s, antibody had been localized to the gamma migrating fraction of electrophoretically separated globular serum proteins[7] (thus, gamma globulin) and a methodology for enriching the concentration of antibody (Cohn fractionation)[8] had been developed. Bruton treated his patients with gamma globulin administered subcutaneously.[1] Bruton also mentioned the use of a spreading factor (hyaluronidase) to facilitate subcutaneous IG (SCIG) administration. Over the next 10 to 15 years, intramuscular administration became the routine in North America and most of

Europe. The pain of intramuscular IG (IMIG) injections restricted the dose, limiting the efficacy. Although IMIG decreased the frequency of invasive infections such as bacteremia, it did not prevent the development of chronic lung disease.

IG therapy was revolutionized when, in late 1981, intravenous IG (IVIG) therapy was approved.[2] With IVIG, the only limitation on the dose was the ability of the patient's heart and kidneys to tolerate the fluid load. The impact of increased doses will be discussed later in this article. In 2014 enzyme facilitated SCIG using recombinant human hyaluronidase to improve bulk fluid flow and bioavailability was approved in the United States.[4]

Since the introduction of IVIG, there has been naming confusion. The 3 major manufacturers used IVIG, IGIV, and IVIg, then SCIG and IGSC. The Food and Drug Administration (FDA) uses IGIV and IGSC. The use of IVIG to refer to all routes of administration should be avoided.

Immunoglobulin Manufacture

IG products available in the United States are made from a pool of at least 1500 (as many as 10–20,000) units of plasma donated in the United States. Plasma is obtained either from outdated units of fresh frozen plasma from volunteer blood donors (recovered plasma) or from paid pheresis donors (source plasma). IgG is initially extracted from the plasma by cold ethanol precipitation or affinity chromatography. The IgG is further purified by one or more additional procedures. Regardless of the origin of the plasma, donations have undergone rigorous testing beginning with the donor questionnaire used for routine blood donation and followed by serologic and DNA testing for blood borne pathogens. The manufacturing process includes at least 3 processes designed to eliminate or inactivate envelop and nonenvelop viruses and prions. An outline of the manufacturing process for IG is shown in **Box 3**. The approach is the same for preparations intended for subcutaneous administration as for IV use. Several IVIG and SCIG products differ only by the final IgG concentration.

In addition to IgM isohemagglutinins, many plasma donors have IgG anti–red blood cell antibodies. If the IgG titer of anti–red cell antibodies is too high, administration may cause hemolysis.[9] When this risk was identified, the FDA instituted release criteria limiting the titer of anti–red blood cell antibodies. Thromboembolic events (TEEs) are serious side effects of IG treatments. One major cause of TEEs has been the presence of activated coagulation factor 11,[10] so manufacturers are now required to limit the activated factor 11 activity. Although activated factor 11 is not the only potential risk factor for thrombosis in PIDD patients, this precaution may decrease the incidence of IG-related TEEs. In addition to safety testing, IG products must meet FDA standards for the presence of sufficient quantities of specific IgG antibodies to rubeola and hepatitis B.

The final steps in IG manufacture are concentration adjustment and packaging as either a liquid or a lyophilized product. The characteristics of IG products are shown in **Box 4**.

Pharmacokinetics of Immunoglobulin G

In order to optimize IG therapy, the prescriber must understand what happens to administered IgG. IgG, whether endogenously produced or infused, ultimately resides 50% within the circulation and 50% in the extravascular, interstitial space. IVIG, initially entirely intravascular, undergoes redistribution and ultimately is catabolized. In contrast, SCIG is initially absorbed, primarily via lymphatics, from the subcutaneous infusion site and then redistributed and finally catabolized. Facilitated SCIG (fSCIG) uses recombinant human hyaluronidase to fragment the hyaluronan that fills the

---

Box 3
Immunoglobulin manufacture

Plasma origin
- Recovered (blood donor)
- Source (pheresis) plasma

Initial extraction
- Cohn fractionation—cold ethanol precipitation
- Affinity chromatography

Additional isolation steps
- Ion exchange chromatography
- Polyethylene glycol precipitation
- Caprylate precipitation

Viral safety
- Low pH exposure
- Trace enzyme exposure
- Pasteurization
- Solvent detergent treatment
- Nanofiltration

Stabilization
- Carbohydrate—mannose, maltose, sucrose
- Saline
- Amphophilic amino acids—glycine, proline

Box 4
Immunoglobulin product characteristics

Storage
- Refrigerated or room temperature

5% IVIG products
- Lyophilized or liquid
- Carbohydrate stabilized (most 5% products)
- Some contain saline

10% IVIG products
- Liquid
- Amino acid stabilized
- Sodium free

Conventional SCIG products—available in 20% and 10% concentrations
- Amino acid stabilized, sodium free

Enzyme-facilitated subcutaneous IG (fSCIG) products
- One 10% product, Sodium free, amino acid–stabilized product using recombinant human hyaluronidase

IgA concentration, osmolality, and pH varies among products

All products have virtually no measurable IgM or IgE

subcutaneous space creating nanometer-sized microchannels that enhance bulk fluid flow. fSCIG follows the same sequence of absorption, redistribution, and catabolism as conventional SCIG but with different characteristics.

Differences in the pharmacokinetics are highlighted in **Fig. 1**. IVIG has a high IgG peak on day one of infusion, with much lower IgG peaks with SCIG and fSCIG. IVIG and fSCIG have identical catabolic phases, but a higher dose of SCIG is needed to maintain comparable IgG trough concentrations. High IgG concentrations are thought to be a risk factor both for serious adverse events such as TEE and for more common but milder infusion side effects such as headache, myalgias, and malaise (see sections on Safety and Tolerability). The bioavailability of IgG, as measured by the area under the time/concentration curve differs for the 3 administration modalities. By definition, the bioavailability of IVIG is 100% because it is all given intravenously. Because SCIG is incompletely absorbed, its bioavailability is 63% relative to IVIG and to achieve bioequivalence with IVIG a 30% to 37% higher dose must be given. fSCIG is 92% bioavailable (considered by FDA to be bioequivalent to IVIG) and is used at the same dose as IVIG. See the section on dosing for a more complete discussion of route of administration and dose.

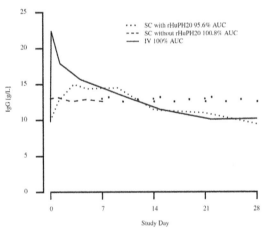

Fig. 1. IGIV and IGHy data at 28-day dosing interval. IVIG (IV) and fSCIG (SC with rHuPH20) data at 28-day dosing interval. SCIG (SC without rHuPH20) data at 7-day dosing interval. Heavy dotted line shows weekly SCIG dose extrapolated over 21 additional days. One hundred eight percent was considered bioequivalent per FDA guidance (interval should fall within a bioequivalence limit, usually 80%–125%). (*From* Wasserman RL, Melamed I, Stein MR, et al. Recombinant human hyaluronidase-facilitated subcutaneous infusion of human immunoglobulins for primary immunodeficiency. J Allergy Clin Immnol 2012;130(4):954; with permission.)

Efficacy

The goal of IG therapy for PIDD is infection prevention. The primary outcome of all pivotal trials of IG products is the rate of acute serious bacterial infections (**Box 5**).

FDA's required rate of acute serious bacterial infections is less than one per patient year, a goal easily met by all products. The secondary efficacy outcomes include all infections and measures that are surrogates for infection, such as days of antibiotic use, days missed from school or work, unscheduled sick visit, and days hospitalized for infection. The rate of all infections in IG licensing trials is about 3 to 4 per patient-year. It is useful to keep this in mind when setting patient expectations for the response to IG therapy.

Box 5
Acute serious bacterial infections
• Bacterial pneumonia
• Bacteremia/sepsis
• Osteomyelitis/septic arthritis
• Bacterial meningitis
• Visceral abscess
The FDA has established specific diagnostic criteria for each of these infections.

Dosing

Since the 1980s there have been several studies confirming that higher IG doses result in better outcomes.[11] A meta-analysis of 17 pivotal trials of IVIG by Orange and colleagues[12] showed an increase in serum IgG concentration of 121 mg/dL for every 100 mg/kg/28 days increase in IVIG dose. The same analysis demonstrated that an increment of 100 mg/dL in IgG concentration resulted in a 27% decrease in the incidence of pneumonia[12] (**Figs. 2** and **3**).

Although these studies support the notion of a relationship between IVIG dose and infection prevention, they do not define the ideal dose. A report by Bonagura and colleagues[13] made the argument that each patient had their own specific dose to achieve the ideal infection prevention. **Fig. 4** shows that patient "a" does well with a trough of 900 mg/dL, whereas patient "b" can be maintained with a trough of 700 mg/dL. More robust support for this notion was provided by the report of Lucas and colleagues[14] showing that while mean trough levels required to achieve low infection rates (≤4.5 per year vs ≤2.5 per year or 0.0 per year) tended to increase as the infection rate decreased, for each infection frequency there were patients with low trough levels and patients with very high trough levels (**Fig. 5**).

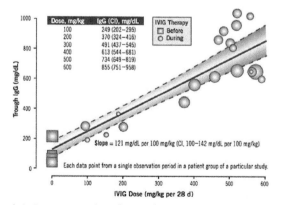

Fig. 2. Mean trough IgG concentrations from subjects participating in pivotal trials of new IVIG products (y-axis) are plotted against IVIG dose per 28 days (x-axis). The size of the circles and squares represents the number of subjects in each study. (*Adapted from* Orange JS, Grossman WJ, Navickis RJ, et al. Impact of trough IgG on pneumonia incidence in primary immunodeficiency: a meta-analysis of clinical studies. Clin Immunol 2010;137(1):26; with permission.)

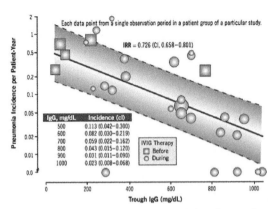

Fig. 3. The incidence of pneumonia per patient-year, validated according to the FDA defini-tion of an acute serious bacterial infection, is plotted on the y-axis against the trough IgG concentration on the x-axis and shows that an increase in the trough IgG concentration of 100 mg/dL decreases the incidence of pneumonia by 27%. (*Adapted from* Orange JS, Grossman WJ, Navickis RJ, et al. Impact of trough IgG on pneumonia incidence in primary immunodeficiency: a meta-analysis of clinical studies. Clin Immunol 2010;137(1):26; with permission.)

Safety—Major Adverse Events

Serious, life-threatening side effects of IG therapy are uncommon in general and rare in PIDD.[15] The risk of major side effects is dose related and the replacement dose for PIDD patients is lower than the immunomodulatory dose. The major, life-threatening side effects of IG therapy and their associated risk factors are shown in **Box 6**. Some of these problems are very rare and idiopathic but there are mitigation strategies to decrease the risk of some adverse reactions (**Box 7**).

Extraction methodology, IgA concentration, minor excipients, and viral safety procedures are not important factors in choosing a particular IG product for most patients. Clinicians should be mindful, however, of the risk factors for major adverse events associated with IG therapy and prescribe accordingly. In addition, for IVIG, the infusion rate is also a risk factor, particularly for thromboembolic events. The relative risk of severe reactions or life-threatening events occurring with SCIG or fSCIG compared with IVIG is unknown. The rate of milder adverse

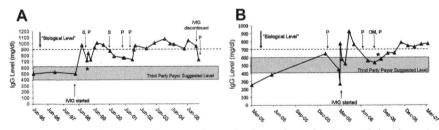

Fig. 4. (*A, B*) Data from 2 patients are shown in these plots of IgG trough levels against time. Infections, otitis media (OM), pneumonia (P), and sinusitis (S) are indicated by arrows. The gray bands indicate the insurance provider's recommended trough IgG levels. (*From* Bonagura VR, Marchlewski R, Cox A, et al. Biologic IgG level in primary immunodeficiency disease: the IgG level that protects against recurrent infection. J Allergy and Clin Immunol 2008;122(1):211; with permission.)

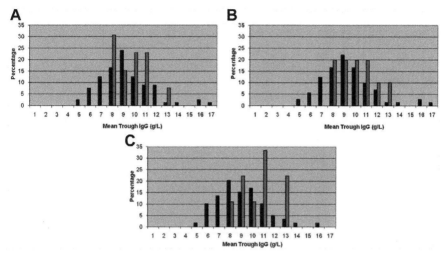

Fig. 5. The mean IgG trough levels of patients with common variable immunodeficiency (red bars) and X-linked agammaglobulinemia (blue bars) during different time periods defined by infection frequency goals of (*A*) ≤ 4.5 per year, (*B*) ≤2.5 per year, and (*C*) 0 per year. (*From* Lucas M, Lee M, Lortan J, et al. Infection outcomes in patients with common variable immunodeficiency disorders: relationship to immunoglobulin therapy over 22 years. J Allergy Clin Immunol 2010;125(6):1357; with permission.)

events, however, is substantially higher with IVIG than with either subcutaneous modality (see later discussion).

Minor adverse reactions are common, occurring in as many as 25% of recipients (**Box 8**). These problems are more frequently seen with IVIG on the first or second infusion or after a hiatus in treatment but may be an ongoing issue. Because there are no trials comparing one product with another, there are no data comparing products based on the reported rate of adverse events. Individual patients may tolerate one product better than another. Differential tolerability is particularly true of intravenously

---

Box 6

Major, life-threatening side effects of IG therapy and their associated risk factors

Renal injury or failure

- Carbohydrate-containing products, particularly sucrose

- Risks—increasing age, renal compromise, diabetes

Thrombosis

- Activated factor 11a contamination

- Risks—increasing age, previous thrombotic event, thrombophilia, hyperviscosity

Hemolysis

- Elevated antibody titers against blood group antigens A and B

Aseptic meningitis

- History of migraine

Transfusion-related lung injury

- No known risk factors

Box 7
Mitigating the risk of immunoglobulin infusions

Age
• Avoid carbohydrate-containing products in the elderly

Comorbid condition risks
• Diabetes or renal disease—avoid carbohydrate-containing products
• Thrombosis history—limit dose per infusion, limit infusion rate
• Cardiac disease—avoid sodium-containing products, use more concentrated products

General risk factors
• Dose per infusion
• Use a lower dose and shorter infusion dose interval
• Decrease the infusion rate
• Although frequently used in the past, it is seldom appropriate to tolerate the risks of an indwelling venous access device solely for IG infusions.

Selection of route of administration: SCIG or fSCIG have lower risk

---

administered IG. Therefore, while IG may be a generic product in terms of efficacy, prescribers should always specify the particular brand of IG to decrease the risk of a patient being exposed to a product that they do not tolerate (**Box 8**).

Mitigation strategies for improving the tolerability of IVIG are often effective. Although these interventions are not sufficient in all cases, pretreatment with glucocorticoids, triptans, or dehydroepiandrosterone may be helpful. Unfortunately, there are no clinical trials demonstrating the efficacy of these pharmacologic interventions (**Box 9**).

Virtually all patients treated with SCIG experience at least one infusion site reaction. In studies of SCIG and fSCIG products, the frequency and severity of these reactions decreased dramatically over the first months of therapy and most patients tolerate SCIG and fSCIG without ongoing difficulties.[3,4,16,17] It is very important for the treating team to educate patients and families before beginning subcutaneous

---

Box 8
Minor systemic adverse events

Most common

• Migraine headache

• Myalgia

• Malaise

• Fatigue

Less common

• Fever

• Diarrhea

• Rash

• Cough

• Chest tightness

• Sinus tenderness

Box 9
Prevention of minor IVIG adverse events

1981 to mid-2000s

- Prehydration with fluids
- Slow the administration rate
- Change the product
- Premedicate with nonsteroidal antiinflammatory drugs (NSAIDs), antihistamine, and/or steroids

After 2005

- Change to SCIG

After 2014

- Change to SCIG or fSCIG

---

therapy because setting appropriate expectations decreases the impact of infusion site reactions and is thought to enhance adherence.[18] Strategies for minimizing the impact of infusion site reactions are shown in **Box 10**. A common cause of site reactions is underestimation of the depth of the subcutaneous space. A longer subcutaneous needle often solves the problem of infusion site reactions. The common practice of priming the infusion set until a drop of fluid is seen at the needle tip should be avoided because subcutaneous needles coated with IgG are more likely to induce pain at the site (**Box 10**).

Although most PIDD patients are able to tolerate any IG replacement product via any mode of administration, there are special populations of patients (**Box 11**) whose conditions influence the choice of a particular IG or route of administration.

Box 10
SCIG and fSCIG adverse event management

Infusion site reactions

- Use a longer needle
- Clean needle tip if IgG solution is visible
- Local heat or cold depending on patient preference
- Change products
- Topical anesthetic
- Topical diphenhydramine
- Topical NSAIDs

Systemic adverse events

- Change products
- Hyper-fractionate the dose (ie, give smaller, more frequent doses)

Adherence—too many needle sticks/infusions per month

- Increase the concentration, decrease infusion frequency
- Change to fSCIG or IVIG

Box 11
Choosing IG products for special populations

- Hemodynamically unstable neonates—10% IVIG, sodium and carbohydrate free
- Compensated congestive heart failure—20% SCIG or 10% sodium and carbohydrate free
- Renal compromise, diabetes, elderly—carbohydrate free
- Poorly controlled migraine—SCIG—or if using IVIG, consider giving only 50% of the planned dose on the first administration
- Hyperviscosity (eg, MGUS)—use 5% or 10% product and a slow infusion rate

Abbreviation: MGUS, monoclonal gammopathy of undetermined significance.

Burden of Care

In addition to the burden of disease suffered by PIDD patients, the burden of care of treatment should not be underestimated. Although it is easy to identify elements of IG treatment that pose a burden to patients and their families, it is not possible to define an ideal approach that will be suitable for every PIDD patient.

Because of the pain of injection and the dosing limitations, IG replacement therapy should not be administered IM. IVIG is typically administered every 3 or 4 weeks in a single infusion that lasts 2 to 4 hours. In most patients, a health care professional starts the IV although the infusion may be given in a physician's office, infusion center, or at home. In contrast, most patients receiving SCIG or fSCIG are treated at home and self-infuse or are assisted by a parent or other trained caregiver. SCIG infusions are usually given weekly but may be administered as often as daily or as infrequently as every 2 weeks. SCIG infusions should last about 1 hour. Most patients self-administer fSCIG or are assisted by a trained parent or other caregiver. Infusions, given every 2, 3, or 4 weeks, should last approximately 2 hours. The features of each route are shown in **Table 1**.

Using the model of shared decision-making will help the practitioner in selecting the product/route of administration that will minimize the burden of care. The major issues that affect most patients are listed in **Box 12**.

A cursory examination of **Box 12** reveals obvious conflicts. The duration of a subcutaneous infusion can be decreased by 50% if the number of infusion sites (ie, needle

---

Table 1
Choosing a mode of administration

	IGIV	Conventional IGSC	fSCIG
Infusion frequency	Every 3–4 wk	Daily to every 2 wk	Every 2–4 wk
Treatment options	Medical supervision Venous access	Self-administration No venous access	Self-administration or HCP No venous access
Location of care	Office, infusion center, home	Home	Office, Infusion Center, Home
Bioavailability	100%	~63%	92%
Relative dose	100%	137% of IV	100%
Sites/month	1	4–20	1–2
Systemic AEs	Higher than IGSC	Lower than IGIV	Similar to IGSC
Local AEs	Lower than IGSC	Higher than IGIV	Similar to IGSC

Abbreviation: AE, adverse event.

Box 12
Burdens of IG therapy

Location of care

- Travel to an infusion center, clinic, or hospital takes time and the added costs of parking and meals away from home.

- Institutional settings are often inefficient adding hours of bureaucracy to the time actually required for infusions.

- Home-based infusions requiring a nurse may be perceived by families as an invasion of privacy.

- Infusions given by a health care provider require advance scheduling that may not be flexible.

Infusion frequency

- Patients generally prefer infrequent infusions, although less frequent infusions may take longer.

Infusion duration

- Published infusion times report the time of the actual IG drug administration.

- Patients consider the infusion time to begin when the drug and equipment is assembled and to end when waste materials are discarded and equipment is put away.

Needle sticks

- Ideally, IV line placement requires a single quick stick.

- Subcutaneous needle placement is easier than starting an IV but is still a needle stick.

- Many children and some adults find all needle sticks very unpleasant.

- Because the penetration of a subcutaneous needle is more superficial than many IVs, topical anesthetics may be more helpful.

---

sticks) is doubled. Similarly, decreasing the dose to minimize minor adverse events will require more frequent dosing. These considerations obligate the clinician to include the patient/parent in a process of shared decision-making when choosing a mode of IG administration. There are, however, circumstances that dictate, at least initially, a specific route for IG therapy. Some of those circumstances are summarized in **Box 13**. Regardless of the route chosen or how that route was selected, it is important to explain to patients that selecting a particular modality is not a life-long decision. As life circumstances change, it may be appropriate to change the way IgG is delivered.

Box 13
Special circumstances influencing the choice of mode of administration

- The patient is hospitalized due to infection: administer 1 g/kg IV over 12 to 24 hours; however, caution is required because IgG may worsen inflammation.

- IVIG or fSCIG in the office or infusion center is the treatment of choice if the patient requires frequent ongoing monitoring because of the severity of the underlying disease or side effects of IG or if the patient/family is unable to self-administer.

- Enzyme-facilitated subcutaneous may be preferred when there is poor venous access and when frequent SCIG infusions are problematic.

- Conventional or facilitated subcutaneous infusion is preferred when systemic adverse events caused by IVIG are significant.

Educating Patients and Families

The primary responsibility for educating PIDD patients and their families about IG therapy rests with the physician. Regardless of the practice setting or support staff available, educational tools are available from the Immune Deficiency Foundation (IDF) and from the individual manufacturers. When discussing IG therapy, the physician explains the features, virtues, and drawbacks of each mode of administration and provides resource materials as well as links to the IDF Website, www.primaryimmune.org. At the same time, the patients are asked to visit the websites of representative IVIG, SCIG, and fSCIG products that explain each process. After this educational process, the patient is asked to meet again to agree on the best initial therapy (**Box 13**).

Ordering Immunoglobulin G Therapy

Despite their ultimate responsibility, physicians seldom need to be engaged with the equipment used for medication delivery. In order to optimize care, physicians should be familiar with the equipment requirements for IG therapy. **Box 14** contains an annotated list of the equipment and supplies used in IG administration.

Because of differences in product tolerability, orders for IG should specify a specific brand. For IVIG therapy the rate ramp up and maximum rate should be specified. For SCIG, orders should include the number of sites, needle length, and infusion rate. Because fSCIG requires a rate ramp up for each

---

Box 14
Hardware for immunoglobulin infusion

IV administration

- Drip with gravity feed and drop counting to determine rate is inexpensive but may be inconsistent
- Standard IV infusion pumps
- Standard IV catheters readily available

Conventional SCIG

- Mechanical, windup syringe pumps: easy to use and often less expensive than other pumps
- Electromechanical syringe or peristaltic pumps: may be used when infusions take too long using mechanical pumps
- Standard IV pumps: may be used for multiple subcutaneous infusion sites but built-in pressure shut-offs may cause problems due to the back pressure in conventional subcutaneous infusion
- 27-gauge infusion sets have been used but more rapid flow rates are better accommodated by 24-gauge thin-walled high-flow needle sets
- Needle length is important and is frequently too short. Multiple needle lengths are available

Enzyme-facilitated SCIG (fSCIG)

- Electromechanical syringe or peristaltic pumps
- Because of the high-flow rates, pumps with high pressure shut-offs are necessary to accommodate the high back pressure in the tubing
- Thin-walled, 24-gauge, high-flow infusion sets are necessary to accommodate the high-flow rate
- Needle length is important: select needle length to reduce site reactions

infusion, that should be specified in addition to the number of sites and maximum infusion rate.

Ensuring Access to Care

Theoretically, if the clinician adheres to the approach discussed in the Indications for IG Therapy section earlier, obtaining payer approval should be routine. The approach outlined in **Box 15** has been effective.

Ongoing Monitoring

The frequency of follow-up visits should be determined by the needs of the individual patient and may be as often as monthly or as infrequently as once a year. The purpose of these visits is to ensure that therapy is adequately efficacious and well tolerated. Questions that should be asked at every visit are listed in **Box 16**.

In addition to follow-up visits, IG recipients should have safety studies, complete blood count and liver and renal function studies, performed at least once a year. IgG concentrations should be monitored no less than once a year. In addition, IgG should be measured before and after changes in dose, product, and modality of administration. Because some immunodeficiencies evolve over time, periodic measurement of IgA and IgM may also be useful.

Future Developments in Immunoglobulin Therapy

Devices to simplify the delivery of SCIG and fSCIG are currently under development and likely to be available soon. At the time of this writing, an IVIG product with high titers of anti–respiratory syncytial virus antibody has been approved and is awaiting commercial release. It is likely that other hyperimmune products are in the pipeline. An alternative approach, also under study, is to spike

---

Box 15
Letters of medical necessity

Authorization letter (letter of medical necessity)
- ICD-10 diagnosis, specific product including J code (for new products include the NDC code as well), dose per infusion, infusion interval
- Brief clinical history
- Laboratory data (for most payers)
  - IgA, IgG, IgM
  - Response to protein and polysaccharide vaccines

Denial—do not write an appeal letter, request a peer-to-peer conference with a Medical Director
- Be prepared with immediate knowledge of the patient's history and laboratory testing
- Note the name and specialty of the medical director. If you suspect that the medical director has a limited experience with primary immunodeficiency and IG, gently, without condescension, provide the key elements of the background of the diagnosis and treatment.

Denial
- Request a peer-to-peer conference with a company allergist/immunologist

Denial
- Request a peer-to-peer conference with an independent allergist/immunologist

Denial
- Briefly summarize your case and email it to several well-known immunologists requesting an opinion
- Submit the replies

Box 16
Questions to ask immunoglobulin recipients at every visit

- Have there been any infections since the last visit? How many courses of antibiotics have been required?
- How long do infusions take?
- Are there any systemic side effects? When do they occur? How long do they last?
- Are there infusion site reactions? How troublesome are they? How long do they last?
- Is there end of cycle deterioration? When does it begin?

---

plasma-derived polyclonal IgG with monoclonal antibodies directed against important pathogens. Efforts to chemically modify IgG molecules to increase their half-life, thereby lengthening the interval between infusions, have been under study for decades.

SUMMARY

IgG replacement therapy transforms the lives of PIDD patients with antibody production defects. The most appropriate dose is the dose that keeps the patient well. The optimal treatment regimen for a PIDD patient is the one that works best for that patient. Clinicians who understand therapeutic IgG and its delivery will be best able to optimize the care of their patients to achieve the best outcomes.

REFERENCES

1. Bruton OC. Agammaglobulinemia. Pediatrics 1952;9:722–8.
2. Ochs HD, Buckley RH, Pirofsky B, et al. Safety and patient acceptability of intravenous immune globulin in 10 percent maltose. Lancet 1980;2:1158–9.
3. Ochs HS, Gupta S, Kiessling P, et al. Safety and efficacy of self-administered subcutaneous immunoglobulin in patients with primary immunodeficiency diseases. J Clin Immunol 2006;26:265–73.
4. Wasserman RL, Melamed I, Stein MR, et al. Recombinant human hyaluronidase-facilitated subcutaneous infusion of human immunoglobulins for primary immunodeficiency. J Allergy Clin Immunol 2012;130:951–7.
5. Orange JS, Ballow M, Stiehm ER, et al. Use and interpretation of diagnostic vaccination in primary immunodeficiency: a working group report of the basic and clinical immunology interest section of the American Academy of Allergy, Asthma & Immunology. J Allergy Clin Immunol 2012;130:S1–24.
6. von Behring E. Serum therapy in therapeutics and medical science. Available at: https://www.nobelprize.org/nobel_prizes/medicine/laureates/1901/behring-lecture.html. Accessed May 6, 2018.
7. Tiselius A. Electrophoresis of serum globulin: electrophoretic analysis of normal and immune sera. Biochem J 1937;31:1464–77.
8. Oncley JL, Melin M, Richert DA, et al. The separation of the antibodies, isoagglutinins, prothrombin, plasminogen and _1-lipoprotein into subfractions of human plasma. J Am Chem Soc 1949;71:541–50.
9. Berg R, Shebl A, Kimber MC, et al. Hemolytic events associated with intravenous immune globulin therapy: a qualitative analysis of 263 cases reported to four manufacturers between 2003 and 2012. Transfusion 2015;55(Suppl 2):S36–46.

10. Dalakas MC, Clark WM. Strokes, thromboembolic events, and IVIg. Neurology 2003;60:1736–7.
11. Pirofsky B. Safety and toxicity of a new serum immunoglobulin G intravenous preparation, IGIV pH 4.25. Rev Infect Dis 1986;S4:S457–63.
12. Orange JS, Grossman WJ, Navickis RJ, et al. Impact of trough IgG on pneumonia incidence in primary immunodeficiency: a meta-analysis of clinical studies. Clin Immunol 2010;137:21–30.
13. Bonagura VR, Marchlewski R, Cox A, et al. Biologic IgG level in primary immuno-deficiency disease: the IgG level that protects against recurrent infection. J Allergy Clin Immunol 2008;122:210–2.
14. Lucas M, Lee M, Lortan J, et al. Infection outcomes in patients with common variable immunodeficiency disorders: relationship to immunoglobulin therapy over 22 years. J Allergy Clin Immunol 2010;125:1354–60.
15. Hefer D, Jaloudi M. Thromboembolic events as an emerging adverse effect during high-dose intravenous immunoglobulin therapy in elderly patients: a case report and discussion of the relevant literature. Ann Hematol 2005;84:411–5.
16. Hagan JB, Fasano MB, Spector S, et al. Efficacy and safety of a new 20% immunoglobulin preparation for subcutaneous administration, IgPro20, in patients with primary immunodeficiency. J Clin Immunol 2010;30(5):734–45.
17. Suez D, Stein M, Gupta S, et al. Efficacy, safety, and pharmacokinetics of a novel human immune globulin subcutaneous, 20 % in patients with primary immunodeficiency diseases in North America. J Clin Immunol 2016;36:700–12.
18. Wasserman RL. Common infusion-related reactions to subcutaneous immunoglobulin therapy: managing patient expectations. Patient Prefer Adherence 2008;2:163–6. Available at: https://www.dovepress.com/common-infusion-related-reactions-to-subcutaneous-immunoglobulin-thera-peer-reviewed-article-PPA. Accessed May 6, 2018.

Update on Advances in Hematopoietic Cell Transplantation for Primary Immunodeficiency Disorders

Oded Shamriz, MD[a,b], Shanmuganathan Chandrakasan, MD[a],*

KEYWORDS

- Hematopoietic stem cell transplantation • Bone marrow transplantation
- Primary immune deficiency • Immune dysregulation • Conditioning

KEY POINTS

- Reduced toxicity conditioning approaches, graft manipulation strategies, and improvement in supportive care have significantly decreased the complications associated with hematopoietic stem cell transplantation (HSCT) and improved the outcome and the availability of HSCT for primary immunodeficiency disorders (PIDDs).
- HSCT is not curative in all PIDDs, understanding the disease pathogenesis and affected cellular components is critical.
- HSCT outcomes for immune dysregulation disorders are currently suboptimal, but likely to improve. The timing of HSCT, control of disease activity with targeted therapies, and anticipating management of autoimmune manifestations post-HSCT are key to a successful outcome.
- In the authors' opinion, a team approach of immunologists and transplant physicians helps to provide optimal care and HSCT outcomes for PIDD.

INTRODUCTION

In 1968, Robert A. Good performed the first allogeneic hematopoietic stem cell transplantation (HSCT) in an infant with severe combined immunodeficiency (SCID). Immunologic reconstitution was achieved, thus opening a doorway into a new era in

Funding: O. Shamriz's position is supported by the Raymond F. Schinazi International Exchange Program, Emory University School of Medicine, Atlanta, GA.. This work is supported by Atlanta Pediatric Scholars Program (APSP) grant K12HD072245 (NICHD Child Health Research Career Development Award Program, NIH) to S. Chandrakasan.
Conflicts of Interest: None.
a Division of Bone Marrow Transplant, Aflac Cancer and Blood Disorders Center, Children's Healthcare of Atlanta, Emory University School of Medicine, 2015 Uppergate Drive, ECC Room 418, Atlanta, GA 30030, USA; b Pediatric Division, Hadassah-Hebrew University Medical Center, Ein-Kerem, POB 12000, Jerusalem, Israel 91120
* Corresponding author.
E-mail address: Shanmuganathan.chandrakasan@emory.edu

Immunol Allergy Clin N Am 39 (2019) 113–128
https://doi.org/10.1016/j.iac.2018.08.003
0889-8561/19/© 2018 Elsevier Inc. All rights reserved.
immunology.theclinics.com

immunology.[1] This famous HSCT is considered to be a milestone in the treatment of primary immunodeficiency disorders (PIDDs). Since then, HSCT for PIDD (PIDD-HSCT) has rapidly evolved, as new reduced-intensity conditioning (RIC) regimens and better patient care have increased success rates.[2] Furthermore, advances in genetics and clinical immunology, such as the introduction of SCID newborn screening (NBS) programs,[3] use of next-generation sequencing, and a better molecular understanding of PIDD,[4] have helped to identify new PIDDs and diagnose and treat more patients in earlier stages of their disease. Accordingly, in the International Union of Immunologic Societies report of 2017, the number of PIDD-related gene errors has increased to 354.[5]

Divided into 2 sections, this review focuses on current advances in PIDD-HSCT. The first section elaborates on general principles of HSCT and the second highlights updates regarding specific PIDD categories.

PART I
Hematopoietic Stem Cell Transplantation for Immunologists: General Principles

Understanding the general principles of HSCT is critical for a good outcome. Although overall and event-free survival rates have been the metrics for HSCT outcome in PIDD, robust donor stem cell engraftment and correction of the underlying immune defect are usually the ultimate goal. Before considering HSCT for a patient with PIDD, the following issues should be considered:

1. Disease: Which cellular compartments are affected and how?
2. Disease activity: Status of infection, autoimmunity, and nutrition.
3. Donor options: What is the hematopoietic stem cell (HSC) source and degree of human leukocyte antigen (HLA) match, and is the graft manipulated or not before transplantation?
4. Conditioning regimen (immune suppression and myeloablation): How much and what agents?
5. Post-HSCT management: Donor chimerism, graft-versus-host disease (GvHD), infection and immune reconstitution.

Considerations Before Hematopoietic Stem Cell Transplantation

Disease
PIDD and immune dysregulation from defects in the lymphohematopoietic compartment are likely to be corrected by HSCT. However, immune abnormalities due to thymic stromal or gastrointestinal (GI) epithelial barrier defects are unlikely to be corrected by HSCT. Thymic stromal defects are thought to be one cause of poor immune reconstitution and poor HSCT outcomes in patients with tetratricopeptide repeat domain 7a (TTC7a) defect.[6] Similarly, patients with nuclear factor-kappa B essential modulator (NEMO) defects have a varying degree of additional epithelial defects leading to recurrent cutaneous and GI inflammation, thus only partial phenotype correction is achieved with HSCT in patients with NEMO with preexisting GI inflammation.[7] **Fig. 1** highlights different compartments that are affected by PIDD and HSCT role in these diseases.

Complement defects can lead to multisystemic autoimmunity and recurrent infections. Excluding C1q (and to a variable extent C4), which is predominantly produced by monocyte-macrophage cells, other complement compounds and their regulatory proteins are mainly synthesized in the liver and other nonhematopoietic lineage-derived cells. Hence, immune abnormalities from C1q is likely to be corrected by HSCT,[8] whereas autoimmunity and susceptibility to recurrent infection from other complement defects are unlikely to be fixed by HSCT.

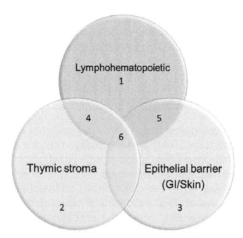

PID category	Lympho-hematopoetic	Thymic stroma	Epithelial Barrier	HSCT outcome	Example
1	+	-	-	Curative	IL2Rγ SCID, CGD
2	-	+	-	Not curative	DiGeorge syndrome, APECED
3	-	-	+	Not curative	Enteropathy from GI barrier defects
4	+	+	-	Partial	
5	+	-	+	Partial	NEMO
6	+	+	+	Partial	TTC7a

Fig. 1. Role of HSCTs in PIDDs affecting different cellular compartments. APECED, autoimmune polyendocrinopathy-candidiasis-ectodermal dystrophy/dysplasia; IL2Rγ, interleukin-2 receptor subunit gamma; PID, primary immune deficiency; +, yes; -, no.

Disease activity and its medical management before hematopoietic stem cell transplantation

Once a decision to proceed to HSCT has been made, optimization of medical management and nutritional rehabilitation is critical for a successful outcome. Aggressive control of infections, autoimmunity, hyperinflammation, and optimization of serum immunoglobulin (Ig)G using immune globulin (IG) replacement is key.

The use of targeted agents, such as abatacept for lipopolysaccharide-responsive and beigelike anchor protein (LRBA) deficiency and cytotoxic T-lymphocyte associated protein 4 (CTLA4) haploinsufficiency,[9] Janus kinase (JAK) inhibitors for signal transducer and activator of transcription (STAT)1 and STAT3 gain-of-function (GOF),[10,11] rapamycin for regulatory T-cell disorders in immune dysregulation, polyendocrinopathy, enteropathy X-linked (IPEX) syndrome,[12] rapamycin or phosphoinositide 3-kinase (PI3k) inhibitor in *PIK3CD* mutations,[13,14] and anakinra for interleukin (IL)-10 and IL-10 receptor (IL-10R) deficiencies,[15] could be used to control disease before HSCT. Better disease control before HSCT has helped decrease the use of broader nonselective agents with higher toxicity, such as glucocorticosteroids and calcineurin inhibitors.

Donor options

Bone marrow has traditionally been the gold standard for HSC source for most pediatric HSCT. However, cord blood and mobilized peripheral blood stem cells (PBSCs) have been variably used in PIDD-HSCT. The use of mobilized PBSC grafts–based haploidentical and unrelated allogeneic HSCT has increased with the availability of graft manipulation approaches to reduce the risk of GvHD that is associated with PBSC grafts. An overview of the different graft sources and their advantages and limitations is highlighted in **Table 1**.

Conditioning regimen: how much and what agents?

In HSCT, conditioning agents are needed for creating bone marrow niche space and for achieving immune suppression to prevent graft rejection. Alkylating chemotherapy or irradiation-based conditioning agents contribute to significant short-term and long-term transplant-related mortality (TRM) and morbidity. The use of reduced toxicity busulfan dosing, treosulfan-based conditioning, and substitution of cyclophosphamide with fludarabine has resulted in decreased toxicity and yet with robust stem cell graft.[16,17] Nonmyeloablative RIC regimens based on melphalan and fludarabine carry reduced TRM risk. However, high incidence of mixed chimerism in this preparative regimen necessitating intensive monitoring and interventions, such as donor lymphocyte infusions (DLI) and HSC boost, might preclude its broader use in PIDD-HSCT.[18] **Table 2** gives an overview of common conditioning agents currently used in PIDD-HSCT.

Several experimental nongenotoxic targeted conditioning approaches are being actively explored. Antibodies targeting CD45 (pan lympho hematopoietic lineage expression) and c-KIT (expressed on hematopoietic stem and progenitor compartment) are being actively investigated to ameliorate the toxicity of chemotherapy or irradiation-based conditioning. Use of anti-CD45 antibody and its radioimmunoconjugate, as a conditioning agent, have shown encouraging results.[19,20] A phase I/II trial, anti-CD45 antibody-based conditioning in 16 patients with PIDD with significant preexisting comorbidities, resulted in full or high-level mixed chimerism in both lymphoid and myeloid lineages in 11 of the 16 patients (69%).[19] Antibody blockade of c-KIT has shown promising results as a conditioning agent in mouse models.[21,22] Conjugation of a cellular toxin to a CD45 antibody has also shown encouraging results in immune-competent murine HSCT models.[23] A phase I clinical trial of a humanized c-KIT antibody, as the conditioning agent, is currently enrolling patients.[24] These nongenotoxic conditioning regimens are badly needed for patients with immune defects due to underlying DNA repair defects (eg, DNA-ligase IV deficiency) which cause decreased tolerance to an alkylating agent or irradiation-based conditioning regimen.

Considerations After Hematopoietic Stem Cell Transplantation

Understanding mixed chimeras

Reduced toxicity conditioning regimens have significantly decreased the TRM associated with PIDD-HSCT; however, with the use of reduced toxicity and RIC regimens there is an increased incidence of mixed chimerism.[16,18] Mixed chimerism in myeloid (CD33) and lymphoid lineage, *often measured in CD3 cells*, has different long-term implications. Myeloid lineage (mainly neutrophils) are short-lived cells in the blood and are dependent on direct bone marrow output; hence, chimerism in the myeloid lineage is usually indicative of donor chimerism in the HSC compartment. Thus, a drop in myeloid chimerism is indicative of donor attrition (graft loss). On the contrary, lymphoid lineage, especially T cells, are long-lived cells, and chimerism in this compartment at the early post-HSCT period may not be reflective of HSC chimerism. In patients with non-SCID PIDD, post-HSCT mixed T-cell chimerism suggests inadequate lymphoablation in the peripheral blood or thymus. In most of the patients with 100% myeloid and mixed T-cell chimerism, the chimerism in the T-cell compartment improves with

Table 1
Hematopoietic stem cell source and its characteristics

HSC Source	Usual Preference	Usual HSC Dose	HLA Match[a]	Limitation	Advances to Overcome Limitations
Bone marrow	Standard, primary graft source in most pediatric HSCT	$3-5 \times 10^6$/kg CD34 ($3-5 \times 10^8$/kg TNC[b])	Usually 10/10 is considered MUD	HSC dose is limited by the amount of bone marrow harvest that can be done safely from a donor	Unmanipulated bone marrow is still considered the gold standard
PBSC (mobilized)	Primary graft in older children where bone marrow cell dose or not adequate, or when graft manipulation is planned	$3-5 \times 10^6$/kg CD34 ($3-5 \times 10^8$/kg TNC)	Usually 10/10 is considered MUD	Higher cGvHD rates	Depletion TCR-α/β+ or CD45RA+ T cells decreases GvHD risk
Cord blood	Ideal of smaller children where adequate HSC dose could be achieved and in viral infection–naive children	$3-5 \times 10^5$/kg[c] CD34	Usually 6/6 is considered matched cord	Limitation in HSC numbers Prolonged neutropenia and delay in immune reconstitution	Double cord or cord blood expansion protocols to overcome limited HSC number

Abbreviations: cGvHD, chronic graft-versus-host disease; HLA, human leukocyte antigen; HSC, hematopoietic stem cells; HSCT, hematopoietic stem cell transplantation; MUD, matched unrelated donor; PBSC, peripheral blood stem cells; TCR, T-cell receptor; TNC, total nucleated cell dose.
  [a] HLA A, B, C, and DRB1-matched is an 8/8 matched donor; HLA A, B, C, DRB1 and DQ-matched is a 10/10 matched donor; HLA A, B, C, DRB1, DQ and DP-matched is a 12/12 matched donor.
  [b] In older teens and young adults with higher body weight, per kg TNC may not be adequate for reduced-intensity preparative regimens.
  [c] Higher dose is usually preferred if greater HLA disparity is noted.

Table 2
Common conditioning regimens for primary immunodeficiency disorder hematopoietic stem cell transplantation

Conditioning Regimens[a]	Myeloablation	Lymphoablation	SOS Risk	Incidence of Mixed Chimerism Myeloid	T Cell
BU/flu	++++	++	++	Low	High
BU/cy	++++	++++	++++	Low	Low
Treo/flu	++++	+++	+	Low	Low
Mel/flu	+++	++++	+	High	Low

Abbreviations: AUC, area under the curve; BU, busulfan; cy, cyclophosphamide; flu, fludarabine; Mel, melphalan; PK, pharmacokinetic; SOS, sinusoidal obstruction syndrome; Treo, treosulfan.
[a] Thiotepa is added to this backbone when additional immune ablation/myelosuppression is desired. However, this adds to alkylator exposure and risk of SOS. BU/flu: BU dose is PK-based reduced toxicity myeloablative AUC range. BU/cy: myeloablative busulfan 16 mg/kg and cyclophosphamide 200 mg/kg total dose. Treo/flu: Standard total doses of treosulfan were 42 g/m^2 or 36 g/m^2. Mel/flu: total dose of melphalan is 140 mg/m^2. Total dose of fludarabine in fludarabine-containing regimens is usually 150 to 180 mg/m^2.

time. Mixed T-cell chimerism during early post-HSCT period may be associated with decreased incidence of GvHD.[16]

Graft-versus-host disease prevention

The donor's naïve T cells, which recognize host major histocompatibility complex antigens, are primarily responsible for GvHD development. Standard-of-care GvHD prophylaxis consists of combined cyclosporine A and short-course methotrexate or mycophenolate mofetil.[25] Post-HSCT cyclophosphamide has been used for GvHD prevention by depleting the alloreactive donor T-lymphocytes responsible for graft rejection and GvHD, while preserving the nonalloreactive memory T cells needed for adaptive immunity and successful engraftment.[26] Post-HSCT cyclophosphamide has largely been used in haploidentical transplants for hematologic malignancies.[27] However, its use in PIDD-HSCT is gaining prominence in developing countries where unrelated donor options are limited and the cost of graft manipulation significant.

Graft manipulation approaches, such as TCR α/β T cells or CD45RA naïve T-cell depletion, are currently being used to decrease GvHD risk.[28,29] α/β T cells are the primary drivers of GvHD, and they represent 90% to 100% of the circulating T-cell population. *Profound* depletion of α/β T cells has been associated with a decreased GvHD rate; the residual γ/δ T cells left in the product after TCR α/β T-cell depletion do not cause GvHD, facilitate engraftment, and offer antiviral immunity.[30,31] Studies using depletion of $\alpha/\beta+$ T cells have documented excellent outcomes with early immune recovery and limited GvHD after haploidentical donor transplantation.[29,32] Thus, with this approach, almost every patient with PIDD can have an excellent HSCT donor option with low GvHD risk.

Management of infection risks

Infections are one of the most common complications after HSCT. Viral infections are of special concern, especially cytomegalovirus (CMV), Epstein-Barr virus (EBV), and adenovirus.[33,34] Unfortunately, the efficacy of treating serious adenovirus infections or preventing EBV-associated posttransplant lymphoproliferative disorder (PTLD) is limited.[35,36] Rituximab, an anti-CD20 monoclonal antibody, is a treatment option for PTLD; however, this medication causes profound B-cell depletion that can persist for up to 6 months or longer.[37]

Both DLI, and virus-specific T-cell therapy (VST) are used for management of active viral infections. Overall, the application of DLI in the treatment of viral infections is limited mostly by its lack of specificity and by the underlying risk of GvHD. Over the past 2 decades, advances made in the development of antigen-specific T-cell therapy have reduced viral infections in the post-HSCT setting.[38] VST products with specificity to multiple viruses, such as EBV, CMV, adenovirus, BK virus, and human herpesvirus-6, have been successfully developed from either donor or third-party T cells. In a retrospective review of 36 patients with primary immune deficiency, who received VST either before or after bone marrow transplantation (BMT), Naik and colleagues[39] demonstrated 81% partial or complete responses against targeted viruses. Their use is currently being evaluated prospectively in a multi-institutional study both before and after HSCT (ClinicalTrials.gov Identifier: NCT03475212).

PART II
Hematopoietic Stem Cell Transplantation for Severe Combined Immunodeficiency

In SCID, early diagnosis and treatment are crucial, as disease course is usually fatal and HSCT at a younger age was found to increase survival rates. NBS through T-cell receptor excision circle analysis has dramatically changed SCID management.[40] Once a diagnosis of SCID is made, HSCT should be done as soon as possible, as overall survival is approximately 90%.[41]

For a long time, the question of pretransplant conditioning for SCID has been contentious. Although unconditioned HSCT using a matched sibling or parental haploidentical donor demonstrated efficacy in improving the survival of critically ill infants with SCID, it is now increasingly apparent that a significant proportion of the long-term survivors have poor long-term naïve T-cell output with features of T-cell exhaustion, a decreasing T-cell repertoire, and poor humoral immune reconstitution necessitating long-term IG replacement.[42,43] In contrast, patients with SCID who received conditioned HSCT have better T-cell and B-cell immune reconstitution with robust naïve T-cell output and a higher rate of independence from IG replacement. This difference was clearly shown in results from 25 North American centers conducting HSCT for SCID in the period of 2000 to 2009.[44]

This difference in the quality of long-term immune reconstitution between conditioned versus unconditioned is likely from the absence of significant HSC engraftment in unconditioned HSCT for SCID resulting in a lack of significant donor B-cell output. Hence, in B + SCID with B-cell–intrinsic defect, such as defects in IL-2Rγ, B-cell class switching defect persists after unconditioned HSCT. This is also apparent in autologous gene therapy trials of IL-2Rγ SCID, in which unconditioned gene therapy resulted in decent T-cell reconstitution but without adequate B-cell reconstitution.[45] Furthermore, conditioned gene therapy and HSCT f or X-SCID resulted in better B-cell reconstitution.[46,47] Although conditioned HSCT for SCID is gaining wider acceptance, the risk of sinusoidal obstruction syndrome (SOS) and long-term comorbidity need to be considered, including busulfan-associated death.[48] In this context, the busulfan dose-deescalation study through the Pediatric Blood and Marrow Transplant Consortium/Primary Immune Deficiency Treatment Consortium could guide us in identifying a safe, yet effective dose to use in these patients. Additionally, the nongenotoxic conditioning approaches highlighted earlier in this review offer exciting possibilities of achieving robust HSC engraftment with minimal genotoxicity.

While considering HSCT for SCID, 2 scenarios warrant additional evaluation. First, in patients with T-B+ SCID, it is essential not to miss thymic defects, such as complete DiGeorge syndrome. In complete DiGeorge syndrome, thymus transplantation rather than HSCT is a more appropriate intervention.[49] Therefore, evaluation for DiGeorge syndrome and intrinsic thymic defects should be considered in these patients before proceeding to HSCT. Second, in patients with T-B− SCID, increased radiation sensitivity (eg, DNA-ligase IV deficiency), which increases the risk of conditioning regimen–associated toxicity and elevates the risk of developing malignancy, should be considered.

Hematopoietic Stem Cell Transplantation for Phagocytic Defects

Phagocytic defects include chronic granulomatous disease (CGD) and leukocyte adhesion defects (LAD). CGD is caused by a defective nicotinamide adenine dinucleotide phosphate (NADPH) oxidase, leading to reduced pathogen killing. Hyperinflammation in CGD is responsible for granuloma formation and inflammatory bowel disease (IBD)-like presentation in some of the patients. This is thought to be due to T-helper (Th)17 and Th1 upregulation and IL-1β overproduction.[50]

HSCT for CGD is widely reported. Conditioning based on reduced toxicity busulfan/fludarabine or treosulfan/fludarabine is becoming the standard for HSCT for CGD. In a seminal multi-institutional HSCT study for CGD, Gungor and colleagues[16] reported at a median follow-up of 21 months, the overall survival was 93% (52 of 56) and event-free survival was 89% (50 of 56). Similar excellent outcomes were noted using treosulfan-based conditioning; this approach was found to be safe and efficient, with more than 90% survival, even in high-risk children with CGD.[51] RIC based on melphalan was found to have a higher rate (75%) of mixed chimerism, hence this is not preferred in most CGD HSCT.[52]

Reports of HSCT in LAD are mainly based on small cohorts. HSCT in LAD-I, the most common type, is reported to be successful using matched family or unrelated donors with varying degrees of GvHD.[53] A cohort of 36 children had good long-term results of HSCT with 28 children receiving myeloablative conditioning and 8 RIC regimens.[54] With increasingly promising results, HSCT, as a curative modality, should be considered in most patients with CGD or LAD-I.

Hematopoietic Stem Cell Transplantation for Primary Immune Deficiency Disorders with Immune Dysregulation

Tregopathies are characterized by immune dysregulation and autoimmunity with underlying quantitative or qualitative defects in T-regulatory cells. A prototype for Tregopathies is IPEX syndrome, which is caused by FOXP3 mutations, resulting in reduced function or number of CD4+ FOXP3+ Treg. Other Tregopathies having an IPEX-like presentation include: LRBA deficiency, STAT1 and STAT3 GOF and CTLA4 haploinsufficiency.[55]

Results of HSCT for Tregopathies are summarized in **Table 3**. HSCT for IPEX has gained acceptance as a curative modality. One study that summarized HSCT results in 58 patients with IPEX from 38 centers showed that survival following HSCT was greater than immunosuppression treatment (73.2 vs 65.1%, respectively). Most reported patients with IPEX have received RIC regimens, and 67% of the patients achieved T-cell reconstitution 1 year following HSCT. But, only 58% (31/53) of the patients achieved full donor chimerism, and even among patients with full donor chimerism only 55% (17/31) were alive and had remission of autoimmunity. Mixed chimerism was noted in 34% (18/53), with disease remission in 50% (9/18). Interestingly, the Treg

Table 3
Hematopoietic stem cell transplantation for IPEX and IPEX-like disorders

Regulatory T-Cell Disorder (Number of Transplanted Patients/Reference)	HSCT Characteristics (% of Transplanted Patients, n)					
	Secondary Graft Failure	Overall Survival	Immune Reconstitution		Patients Who Needed Repeated HSCT	Post-HSCT Resolution of Immune Dysregulation-Related Symptoms
			T-Cell Reconstitution	IVIG Independence		
IPEX (58/Barzaghi et al,[56] 2018)	3.4 (2)	74.1(43)	37.9(22)	51.7 (30)	12.1 (7)	46.5 (27)
IPEX-like STAT1 GOF (15/Leiding et al,[57] 2018)	40 (6)	40 (6)	26.7(4)	26.7 (4)	20 (3)	26.6 (4)
LRBA protein deficiency (12/Seidel et al,[58] 2018)	16.7(2)	66.7(8)	N/A	50 (6)[a]	0 (0)	66.7 (8)[b]
CTLA4 deficiency (8/Slatter et al,[59] 2016)	0 (0)	75 (6)	N/A	75 (6)	0 (0)	87.5 (7)[c]

Abbreviations: CTLA, cytotoxic T-lymphocyte-associated protein; GOF, gain-of-function; HSCT, hematopoietic stem cell transplantation; IPEX, immune dysregulation, polyendocrinopathy, enteropathy, X-linked syndrome; IVIG, intravenous immunoglobulin; LRBA, lipopolysaccharide-responsive beigelike anchor; N/A, data are not available; STAT, signal transducer and activator of transcription.
  [a] Data are not available in 4 of 12 patients.
  [b] Complete remission and partial remission with and without the need for additional immunosuppressive treatment was noted in 4, 2, and 2 patients, respectively.
  [c] Clinical resolution did not include reversal of type 1 diabetes mellitus.

cells were 100% of donor origin in 3 of 9 patients with mixed chimerism in remission, suggesting survival advantage of donor Treg compartment.[56]

Similar to IPEX, there are several challenges in HSCT for IPEX-like diseases. Experience in HSCT in 15 patients with STAT1 GOF demonstrates low survival rates (40%) and high rates of secondary graft failure (50% of 12 that primarily engrafted).[57] Although these results do not preclude offering HSCT for these patients, further understanding the biology behind high rejection and better disease control to reduce TRM are needed before offering HSCT. Similarly, LRBA deficiency results in decreased CTLA4 expression on the cell surface.[9] Evidence for successful HSCT for LRBA deficiency is accumulating. Seidel and colleagues[58] summarized 12 transplanted LRBA-deficient patients. Survival rate of 67% and high prevalence of patients with symptoms in remission in the 24-month follow-up period were demonstrated. Notably, resolution of enteropathy and cytopenia were noted in most of the CTLA4-deficient patients following HSCT, although HSCT did not reverse the development of type 1 diabetes mellitus.[59]

Patients with IPEX and IPEX-like syndrome are known to have hypergammaglobulinemia and high titers of autoantibodies.[55] In one study, harmonin and villin autoantibodies were identified in 12 and 6 of 13 patients with IPEX. Autoantibody titers were decreased post-HSCT in most patients with IPEX.[60] Therefore, autoantibody titer monitoring may be useful in the long-term follow-up of transplanted patients with IPEX.

Finally, in several Tregopathies, the autoimmune manifestations might take a long time to improve despite complete donor chimerism in peripheral blood. This is likely due to a dysregulated tissue-based immune compartment. Depending on the intensity of conditioning, plasma cell and tissue-based immune compartments can be resistant to the conditioning agents that can still drive autoimmune manifestations post-HSCT. Thus, overall HSCT outcome for Tregopathies is poorer than classic PIDD, such as SCID or CGD. Further research into the biology of these disorders, optimal use of biologicals as a bridge to HSCT, focus on aggressive disease control before HSCT and early referral to HSCT before development of end-organ damage could improve the outcome of these disorders.

Hematopoietic Stem Cell Transplantation for Very Early Onset Inflammatory Bowel Disease

Based on the age of onset, pediatric IBD is categorized as early onset (before the age of 10 years), very early onset (VEO-IBD; before the age of 6 years), and infantile IBD (before the age of 2 years).[61] The younger the onset age, the more likely the disease is monogenic. Monogenic etiology of VEO-IBD is estimated to be 20% to 30%, underscoring the need for genetic testing.[62] Indications for HSCT vary based on underlying defect (**Table 4**).

Of the VEO-IBD group, the most studied are IL-10 and IL-10R deficiencies. IL-10 is an important anti-inflammatory cytokine and chronic inflammation of the bowel in these patients is often hard to control and may require surgical interventions, such as total colectomy and ileostomy.[63] Experience of HSCT in IL-10 and IL-10R–deficient patients shows overall good survival rates and curative results and is increasingly considered the standard of care. In one study, 40 patients with VEO-IBD screened for *IL-10* and *IL-10R* gene mutations, 7 of the patients were identified as IL-10 or IL-10R–deficient, 3 were treated with HSCT and clinically improved.[64] A recent study has recommended postponing surgical intervention and proceeding directly to HSCT, thus achieving clinical remission without the complications of colectomy.[65]

Table 4		
Hematopoietic stem cell transplantations for monogenetic inflammatory bowel diseases		
	Indication for HSCT[a]	Primary Immune Deficiency with IBD
Definitive	Standard of care	IL-10R, IL-10, IPEX, CGD, SCID, WAS
Variable	HSCT is likely to curative, might have higher complications	STAT3 GOF, LRBA, CTLA4, XIAP[b] NEMO,[c] STAT1 GOF
Unlikely to help	HSCT is not likely to help and will cause more harm than good	TTC7a[d] and other epithelial barrier defects

Abbreviations: CGD, chronic granulomatous disease; CTLA4, cytotoxic T-cell lymphocyte antigen; GOF, gain-of-function; LRBA, lipopolysaccharide-responsive beigelike anchor; HSCT, hematopoietic stem cell transplantation; IL-10R, interleukin-10 receptor; IPEX, immune dysregulation, polyendocrinopathy, enteropathy, X-linked; NEMO, nuclear factor-kappa B essential modulator; SCID, severe combined immune deficiency; STAT, signal transducer and activator; TTC7a, tetratricopeptide repeat domain-7a; WAS, Wiskott-Aldrich syndrome; XIAP, X-linked inhibitor of apoptosis protein.
[a] The role of HSCT is decided based on standard matched sibling and matched unrelated HSCT outcomes.
[b] High mortality rates with myeloablative conditioning.[71]
[c] Experimental models and reports suggest there could be worsening of colitis after HSCT. However, there are reports of patients with complete immune reconstitution and no worsening of colitis after HSCT.[7]
[d] HSCT has been done in some patients to correct underlying SCID.[6]

As the baseline state of patients with VEO-IBD consists of chronic GI inflammation, risk for gut GvHD is potentially high. Therefore, controlling GI inflammation in transplanted patients with VEO-IBD is the key, and transition of biologicals during HSCT should be carefully tailored and monitored to avoid IBD exacerbation.

Hematopoietic Stem Cell Transplantation for Autoinflammatory and Hyperinflammatory Disorders

The defects in the inflammasome pathway cause excess production of IL-1β and IL-18, resulting in hyperinflammation.[66,67] Inflammasome defects in which HSCT has been performed include familial Mediterranean fever (FMF), hyper IgD syndrome, systemic-onset juvenile idiopathic arthritis (SJIA), and X-linked inhibitor of apoptosis protein (XIAP) deficiency.

Reports of HSCT for FMF are sporadic. Milledge and colleagues[68] reported 1 patient presenting with both congenital dyserythropoietic anemia and FMF. HSCT, performed at 4 years of age, resulted in complete resolution of FMF symptoms during 2 years of follow-up. However, questions regarding the role of HSCT in curing FMF in this patient remain unanswered, and HSCT is currently not standard of care for FMF.[69,70] XIAP commonly presents with either hemophagocytic lymphohistiocytosis (HLH) or refractory IBD. An international study of 19 patients revealed that overall survival was low (14%) in patients with XIAP receiving myeloablative conditioning, as compared with RIC (55%). Most deaths in this study were related to SOS. Therefore, myeloablative conditioning is not recommended for HSCT in patients with XIAP.[71] Furthermore, management of HLH before and after HSCT requires attention, as it affects overall HSCT outcomes.[71]

In SJIA, most have no monogenetic defects and are complicated by debilitating arthritis and recurrent life-threatening macrophage-activating syndrome. In a multicenter study, 11 patients with SJIA and 5 patients with polyarticular JIA were transplanted using alemtuzumab and fludarabine-based RIC regimens. Of the 16 patients, 14 survived with improvement in arthritis and HLH.[72] Plasma levels of several cytokines, including IL-18, tumor necrosis factor-α, and macrophage inhibitory factor, were found to be elevated in JIA, suggesting that they are useful in post-HSCT long-term monitoring.[73]

SUMMARY

Clinical immunology and transplant medicine are rapidly evolving. The decision of whether to do HSCT in patients with PIDD should take into account disease-specific considerations. Genetic diagnosis, understanding specific immune abnormalities, aggressive medical management of infectious and noninfectious complications, utilization of current advances in HSCT, such as graft manipulation and reduced toxicity conditioning agents, and continued teamwork between immunologists and transplant physicians before and after HSCT hold the key for a successful HSCT in these patients.

REFERENCES

1. Ballow M. Historical perspectives in the diagnosis and treatment of primary immune deficiencies. Clin Rev Allergy Immunol 2014;46(2):101–3.
2. Kapoor N, Raj R. Hematopoietic stem cell transplantation for primary immune deficiency disorders. Indian J Pediatr 2016;83(5):450–4.
3. King JR, Hammarstrom L. Newborn screening for primary immunodeficiency diseases: history, current and future practice. J Clin Immunol 2018;38(1):56–66.
4. Heimall JR, Hagin D, Hajjar J, et al. Use of genetic testing for primary immunodeficiency patients. J Clin Immunol 2018;38(3):320–9.
5. Picard C, Bobby Gaspar H, Al-Herz W, et al. International Union of Immunological Societies: 2017 primary immunodeficiency diseases committee report on inborn errors of immunity. J Clin Immunol 2018;38(1):96–128.
6. Kammermeier J, Lucchini G, Pai SY, et al. Stem cell transplantation for tetratricopeptide repeat domain 7A deficiency: long-term follow-up. Blood 2016;128(9):1306–8.
7. Miot C, Imai K, Imai C, et al. Hematopoietic stem cell transplantation in 29 patients hemizygous for hypomorphic IKBKG/NEMO mutations. Blood 2017;130(12):1456–67.
8. Olsson RF, Hagelberg S, Schiller B, et al. Allogeneic hematopoietic stem cell transplantation in the treatment of human c1q deficiency: the Karolinska experience. Transplantation 2016;100(6):1356–62.
9. Lo B, Zhang K, Lu W, et al. Autoimmune disease. Patients with LRBA deficiency show CTLA4 loss and immune dysregulation responsive to abatacept therapy. Science 2015;349(6246):436–40.
10. Weinacht KG, Charbonnier LM, Alroqi F, et al. Ruxolitinib reverses dysregulated T helper cell responses and controls autoimmunity caused by a novel signal transducer and activator of transcription 1 (STAT1) gain-of-function mutation. J Allergy Clin Immunol 2017;139(5):1629–40.e2.
11. 2017 LASID meeting abstracts. J Clin Immunol 2017;1–74.
12. Yong PL, Russo P, Sullivan KE. Use of sirolimus in IPEX and IPEX-like children. J Clin Immunol 2008;28(5):581–7.
13. Maccari ME, Abolhassani H, Aghamohammadi A, et al. Disease evolution and response to rapamycin in activated phosphoinositide 3-kinase delta syndrome: the European Society for Immunodeficiencies-Activated Phosphoinositide 3-Kinase delta Syndrome Registry. Front Immunol 2018;9:543.

14. Rao VK, Webster S, Dalm V, et al. Effective "activated PI3Kdelta syndrome"-targeted therapy with the PI3Kdelta inhibitor leniolisib. Blood 2017;130(21): 2307–16.
15. Shouval DS, Biswas A, Kang YH, et al. Interleukin 1beta mediates intestinal inflammation in mice and patients with interleukin 10 receptor deficiency. Gastroenterology 2016;151(6):1100–4.
16. Gungor T, Teira P, Slatter M, et al. Reduced-intensity conditioning and HLA-matched haemopoietic stem-cell transplantation in patients with chronic granulomatous disease: a prospective multicentre study. Lancet 2014;383(9915): 436–48.
17. Slatter MA, Rao K, Amrolia P, et al. Treosulfan-based conditioning regimens for hematopoietic stem cell transplantation in children with primary immunodeficiency: United Kingdom experience. Blood 2011;117(16):4367–75.
18. Marsh RA, Rao MB, Gefen A, et al. Experience with alemtuzumab, fludarabine, and melphalan reduced-intensity conditioning hematopoietic cell transplantation in patients with nonmalignant diseases reveals good outcomes and that the risk of mixed chimerism depends on underlying disease, stem cell source, and alemtuzumab regimen. Biol Blood Marrow Transplant 2015;21(8):1460–70.
19. Straathof KC, Rao K, Eyrich M, et al. Haemopoietic stem-cell transplantation with antibody-based minimal-intensity conditioning: a phase 1/2 study. Lancet 2009; 374(9693):912–20.
20. Mawad R, Gooley TA, Rajendran JG, et al. Radiolabeled anti-CD45 antibody with reduced-intensity conditioning and allogeneic transplantation for younger patients with advanced acute myeloid leukemia or myelodysplastic syndrome. Biol Blood Marrow Transplant 2014;20(9):1363–8.
21. Czechowicz A, Kraft D, Weissman IL, et al. Efficient transplantation via antibody-based clearance of hematopoietic stem cell niches. Science 2007;318(5854): 1296–9.
22. Chandrakasan S, Jayavaradhan R, Ernst J, et al. KIT blockade is sufficient for donor hematopoietic stem cell engraftment in Fanconi anemia mice. Blood 2017;129(8):1048–52.
23. Palchaudhuri R, Saez B, Hoggatt J, et al. Non-genotoxic conditioning for hematopoietic stem cell transplantation using a hematopoietic-cell-specific internalizing immunotoxin. Nat Biotechnol 2016;34(7):738–45.
24. Shizuru JA. AMG191 conditioning/CD34+CD90 stem cell transplant study for SCID patients. 2016. Available at: https://clinicaltrials.gov/ct2/show/NCT02963064. Accessed November 15, 2016.
25. Locatelli F, Bruno B, Zecca M, et al. Cyclosporin A and short-term methotrexate versus cyclosporin A as graft versus host disease prophylaxis in patients with severe aplastic anemia given allogeneic bone marrow transplantation from an HLA-identical sibling: results of a GITMO/EBMT randomized trial. Blood 2000;96(5): 1690–7.
26. Luznik L, Fuchs EJ. High-dose, post-transplantation cyclophosphamide to promote graft-host tolerance after allogeneic hematopoietic stem cell transplantation. Immunol Res 2010;47(1–3):65–77.
27. Robinson TM, O'Donnell PV, Fuchs EJ, et al. Haploidentical bone marrow and stem cell transplantation: experience with post-transplantation cyclophosphamide. Semin Hematol 2016;53(2):90–7.
28. Teschner D, Distler E, Wehler D, et al. Depletion of naive T cells using clinical grade magnetic CD45RA beads: a new approach for GVHD prophylaxis. Bone Marrow Transplant 2014;49(1):138–44.

29. Bertaina A, Merli P, Rutella S, et al. HLA-haploidentical stem cell transplantation after removal of αβ+ T and B cells in children with nonmalignant disorders. Blood 2014;124(5):822–6.

30. Daniele N, Scerpa M, Caniglia M, et al. Transplantation in the onco-hematology field: focus on the manipulation of αβ and γδ T cells. Pathol Res Pract 2012; 208(2):67–73.

31. Locatelli F, Bauquet A, Palumbo G, et al. Negative depletion of α/β+ T cells and of CD19+ B lymphocytes: a novel frontier to optimize the effect of innate immunity in HLA-mismatched hematopoietic stem cell transplantation. Immunol Lett 2013; 155(1–2):21–3.

32. Shah RM, Elfeky R, Nademi Z, et al. T-cell receptor alphabeta(+) and CD19(+) cell-depleted haploidentical and mismatched hematopoietic stem cell transplantation in primary immune deficiency. J Allergy Clin Immunol 2018;141(4): 1417–26.e1.

33. Shields AF, Hackman RC, Fife KH, et al. Adenovirus infections in patients undergoing bone-marrow transplantation. N Engl J Med 1985;312(9):529–33.

34. Gerritsen EJ, Stam ED, Hermans J, et al. Risk factors for developing EBV-related B cell lymphoproliferative disorders (BLPD) after non-HLA-identical BMT in children. Bone Marrow Transplant 1996;18(2):377–82.

35. Tomblyn M, Chiller T, Einsele H, et al. Guidelines for preventing infectious complications among hematopoietic cell transplantation recipients: a global perspective. Biol Blood Marrow Transplant 2009;15(10):1143–238.

36. Yusuf U, Hale GA, Carr J, et al. Cidofovir for the treatment of adenoviral infection in pediatric hematopoietic stem cell transplant patients. Transplantation 2006; 81(10):1398–404.

37. Faye A, Quartier P, Reguerre Y, et al. Chimaeric anti-CD20 monoclonal antibody (rituximab) in post-transplant B-lymphoproliferative disorder following stem cell transplantation in children. Br J Haematol 2001;115(1):112–8.

38. Bollard CM, Heslop HE. T cells for viral infections after allogeneic hematopoietic stem cell transplant. Blood 2016;127(26):3331–40.

39. Naik S, Nicholas SK, Martinez CA, et al. Adoptive immunotherapy for primary immunodeficiency disorders with virus-specific T lymphocytes. J Allergy Clin Immunol 2016;137(5):1498–505.e1.

40. Thakar MS, Hintermeyer MK, Gries MG, et al. A practical approach to newborn screening for severe combined immunodeficiency using the T cell receptor excision circle assay. Front Immunol 2017;8:1470.

41. Heimall J, Buckley RH, Puck J, et al. Recommendations for screening and management of late effects in patients with severe combined immunodeficiency after allogenic hematopoietic cell transplantation: a consensus statement from the second pediatric blood and marrow transplant consortium international conference on late effects after pediatric HCT. Biol Blood Marrow Transplant 2017; 23(8):1229–40.

42. Sarzotti-Kelsoe M, Win CM, Parrott RE, et al. Thymic output, T-cell diversity, and T-cell function in long-term human SCID chimeras. Blood 2009;114(7):1445–53.

43. Buckley RH, Win CM, Moser BK, et al. Post-transplantation B cell function in different molecular types of SCID. J Clin Immunol 2013;33(1):96–110.

44. Pai SY, Cowan MJ. Stem cell transplantation for primary immunodeficiency diseases: the North American experience. Curr Opin Allergy Clin Immunol 2014; 14(6):521–6.

45. Hacein-Bey-Abina S, Pai SY, Gaspar HB, et al. A modified gamma-retrovirus vector for X-linked severe combined immunodeficiency. N Engl J Med 2014;371(15): 1407–17.
46. Miggelbrink AM, Logan BR, Buckley RH, et al. B cell differentiation and IL-21 response in IL2RG/JAK3 SCID patients after hematopoietic stem cell transplantation. Blood 2018;131(26):2967–77.
47. De Ravin SS, Wu X, Moir S, et al. Lentiviral hematopoietic stem cell gene therapy for X-linked severe combined immunodeficiency. Sci Transl Med 2016;8(335): 335ra357.
48. Heimall J, Logan BR, Cowan MJ, et al. Immune reconstitution and survival of 100 SCID patients post-hematopoietic cell transplant: a PIDTC natural history study. Blood 2017;130(25):2718–27.
49. Davies EG, Cheung M, Gilmour K, et al. Thymus transplantation for complete DiGeorge syndrome: European experience. J Allergy Clin Immunol 2017;140(6): 1660–70.e6.
50. Rieber N, Hector A, Kuijpers T, et al. Current concepts of hyperinflammation in chronic granulomatous disease. Clin Dev Immunol 2012;2012:252460.
51. Morillo-Gutierrez B, Beier R, Rao K, et al. Treosulfan-based conditioning for allogeneic HSCT in children with chronic granulomatous disease: a multicenter experience. Blood 2016;128(3):440–8.
52. Khandelwal P, Bleesing JJ, Davies SM, et al. A single-center experience comparing alemtuzumab, fludarabine, and melphalan reduced-intensity conditioning with myeloablative busulfan, cyclophosphamide, and antithymocyte globulin for chronic granulomatous disease. Biol Blood Marrow Transplant 2016; 22(11):2011–8.
53. Al-Dhekri H, Al-Mousa H, Ayas M, et al. Allogeneic hematopoietic stem cell transplantation in leukocyte adhesion deficiency type 1: a single center experience. Biol Blood Marrow Transplant 2011;17(8):1245–9.
54. Qasim W, Cavazzana-Calvo M, Davies EG, et al. Allogeneic hematopoietic stem-cell transplantation for leukocyte adhesion deficiency. Pediatrics 2009;123(3): 836–40.
55. Verbsky JW, Chatila TA. Immune dysregulation, polyendocrinopathy, enteropathy, X-linked (IPEX) and IPEX-related disorders: an evolving web of heritable autoimmune diseases. Curr Opin Pediatr 2013;25(6):708–14.
56. Barzaghi F, Amaya Hernandez LC, Neven B, et al. Long-term follow-up of IPEX syndrome patients after different therapeutic strategies: an international multicenter retrospective study. J Allergy Clin Immunol 2018;141(3):1036–49.e5.
57. Leiding JW, Okada S, Hagin D, et al. Hematopoietic stem cell transplantation in patients with gain-of-function signal transducer and activator of transcription 1 mutations. J Allergy Clin Immunol 2018;141(2):704–17.e5.
58. Seidel MG, Bohm K, Dogu F, et al. Treatment of severe forms of LPS-responsive beige-like anchor protein deficiency with allogeneic hematopoietic stem cell transplantation. J Allergy Clin Immunol 2018;141(2):770–5.e1.
59. Slatter MA, Engelhardt KR, Burroughs LM, et al. Hematopoietic stem cell transplantation for CTLA4 deficiency. J Allergy Clin Immunol 2016;138(2):615–619 e611.
60. Lampasona V, Passerini L, Barzaghi F, et al. Autoantibodies to harmonin and villin are diagnostic markers in children with IPEX syndrome. PLoS One 2013;8(11): e78664.
61. Snapper SB. Very-early-onset inflammatory bowel disease. Gastroenterol Hepatol (N Y) 2015;11(8):554–6.

62. Charbit-Henrion F, Parlato M, Hanein S, et al. Diagnostic yield of next-generation sequencing in very early-onset inflammatory bowel diseases: a multicenter study. J Crohns Colitis 2018;12(9):1104–12.

63. Zhu L, Shi T, Zhong C, et al. IL-10 and IL-10 receptor mutations in very early onset inflammatory bowel disease. Gastroenterology Res 2017;10(2):65–9.

64. Engelhardt KR, Shah N, Faizura-Yeop I, et al. Clinical outcome in IL-10- and IL-10 receptor-deficient patients with or without hematopoietic stem cell transplantation. J Allergy Clin Immunol 2013;131(3):825–30.

65. Kocacik Uygun DF, Uygun V, Daloglu H, et al. Hematopoietic stem cell transplantation from unrelated donors in 2 cases of interleukin-10 receptor deficiency: is surgery not a requirement? J Pediatr Hematol Oncol 2018. [Epub ahead of print].

66. Manthiram K, Zhou Q, Aksentijevich I, et al. The monogenic autoinflammatory diseases define new pathways in human innate immunity and inflammation. Nat Immunol 2017;18(8):832–42.

67. Manthiram K, Zhou Q, Aksentijevich I, et al. Corrigendum: The monogenic autoinflammatory diseases define new pathways in human innate immunity and inflammation. Nat Immunol 2017;18(11):1271.

68. Milledge J, Shaw PJ, Mansour A, et al. Allogeneic bone marrow transplantation: cure for familial Mediterranean fever. Blood 2002;100(3):774–7.

69. Touitou I. Should patients with FMF undergo BMT? Blood 2003;101(3):1205 [author reply: 1205–6].

70. Touitou I, Ben-Chetrit E, Gershoni-Baruch R, et al. Allogenic bone marrow transplantation: not a treatment yet for familial Mediterranean fever. Blood 2003;102(1):409.

71. Marsh RA, Rao K, Satwani P, et al. Allogeneic hematopoietic cell transplantation for XIAP deficiency: an international survey reveals poor outcomes. Blood 2013;121(6):877–83.

72. M F Silva J, Ladomenou F, Carpenter B, et al. Allogeneic hematopoietic stem cell transplantation for severe, refractory juvenile idiopathic arthritis. Blood Adv 2018;2(7):777–86.

73. de Jager W, Hoppenreijs EP, Wulffraat NM, et al. Blood and synovial fluid cytokine signatures in patients with juvenile idiopathic arthritis: a cross-sectional study. Ann Rheum Dis 2007;66(5):589–98.

Genetic Testing to Diagnose Primary Immunodeficiency Disorders and to Identify Targeted Therapy

Jennifer Heimall, MD

KEYWORDS

- Primary immunodeficiency • Chromosomal microarray • Sanger sequencing
- Next-generation sequencing • Whole exome sequencing
- Whole genome sequencing • Gene therapy • Gene editing

KEY POINTS

- There has been a rapid expansion in the number of genetically defined forms of immuno-deficiency or immune dysregulation in the last 10 years.
- Genetic testing helps elucidate the molecular pathways that are disrupted in patients with immunodeficiency.
- Knowledge of the underlying molecular pathway allows for the design of personalized therapy.

INTRODUCTION: HISTORY OF GENETICS IN PRIMARY IMMUNODEFICIENCY

Primary immunodeficiency disorders (PIDDs) generally manifest as increased susceptibility to infection, with certain types of infections classically associated with specific defects of innate or adaptive immunity. Among the early described PIDDs was the clinical description of Bruton agammaglobulinemia. Nearly half a century later, in the 1990s, the mutations in the *BTK* gene were described as the molecular cause of X-linked agammaglobulinemia.[1] The early years of genetic testing focused on diseases with clear patterns of inheritance and high lethality, such as X-linked severe combined immunodeficiency (SCID)[2] and Wiskott Aldrich syndrome (WAS).[3] As molecular techniques evolved and became more accessible for both research and clinical applications, the spectrum of patients with symptoms of immunodeficiency broadened tremendously. It is now well-recognized that molecular defects associated with immune cell dysfunction can lead to symptoms beyond increased susceptibility

Allergy/Immunology, Perelman School of Medicine at University of Pennsylvania, The Children's Hospital of Philadelphia, 3401 Civic Center Boulevard, Philadelphia, PA 19104, USA
E-mail address: heimallj@email.chop.edu

Immunol Allergy Clin N Am 39 (2019) 129–140
https://doi.org/10.1016/j.iac.2018.08.009   immunology.theclinics.com
0889-8561/19/© 2018 Elsevier Inc. All rights reserved.

to infection, including symptoms of autoimmunity, atopy, and autoinflammation. In addition, recent years have brought reports of gain-of-function mutations causing these symptoms, whereas, in the past, the predominant focus was on mutations causing absence or decreased function of the encoded protein. Overall, the number of genetically defined forms of primary immunodeficiency has demonstrated rapid growth in recent years[4] (**Fig. 1**). The latest International Union of Immunologic Societies report, published in early 2018, listed 354 inborn errors of immune function.[4] This reflects increased recognition of the varied phenotypes associated with immune dysfunction, as well as increased availability of whole exome sequencing (WES) and, in some cases, whole genome sequencing (WGS). This article reviews the benefits and limitations of genetic testing for PIDDs and provides a brief overview of the currently available forms of genetic testing. It also explains how treatment decisions can be informed by the results of genetic testing and discusses what implications genetic testing might hold in the future for the management and diagnosis of PIDDs.

BENEFITS OF GENETIC TESTING FOR PRIMARY IMMUNODEFICIENCY

The clinical use of genetic testing in patients with symptoms of immunodeficiency allows for a definitive diagnosis to aid in determination of treatment and in the understanding of prognosis and the risk of recurrence of disease within the family.

The advent of T-cell receptor excision circles (TRECs) measurement for population-based newborn screening (itself a genetic test), has led to a marked increase in the early identification of infants with T-cell deficiency. Although it is of benefit to diagnose and provide hematopoietic stem cell transplant (HSCT) to patients with SCID early in life and before the development of infections,[5] not all of the patients with isolated T-cell deficiency identified via TRECs screening have SCID.[6] A significant subpopulation of these patients has other syndromes associated with T-cell deficiency. In infants with an isolated T-cell deficiency, it is important to consider, through genetic testing, the diagnosis of 22q11 deletion syndrome, or other forms of thymus dysfunction or athymia. This has important treatment ramifications because, although the most common treatment for SCID currently is HSCT, thymus transplant is the recommended treatment for patients with congenital absence of the thymus. Genetic testing can

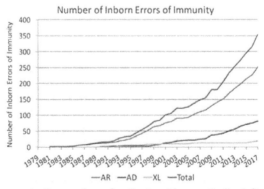

Fig. 1. Marked increase in the number of patients with genetically defined forms of immunodeficiency since 1981, with a particularly steep rate of increase since the introduction of next-generation sequencing. AD, autosomal dominant; AR, autosomal recessive; XL, x-linked. (*From* Picard C, Gaspar HB, Al-Herz W, et al. International Union of Immunological Societies: 2017 primary immunodeficiency diseases committee report on inborn errors of immunity. J Clin Immunol 2018;38(1):97; with permission.)

also inform decisions regarding the use of particular pharmacologic interventions for PIDDs. Increasingly, monogenic causes of immune dysregulation associated with dysfunctional cell signaling have been described. This allows for targeted treatment of the underlying molecular defect using monoclonal antibody-based biologics.

The underlying genetic diagnosis can also aid in prognostication of disease severity and overall clinical outcome. One example is the association of genotype with long-term survival in patients with chronic granulomatous disease (CGD). The X-linked form of CGD tends to be associated with lower residual oxidative capacity and, therefore, has a more severe clinical course than the autosomal recessive (AR) CGD genotypes, with significant differences in age at diagnosis and mean survival age.[7,8] Other correlations between genetics and prognosis include the impact of deletion size on T-cell counts in patients with 22q11 deletion syndrome[9]; the impact of site of the specific mutation within the *MEFV*, *MVK*, *TNFRSF1A*, and *NLRP3* genes on symptoms and likely treatment responsiveness[10]; and the correlation of *RAG2* mutations with recombination activity and severity of disease symptoms.[11]

Finally, knowledge of the pattern of inheritance of disease empowers patients and their families to know their risk of recurrence of disease. In vitro fertilization paired with preimplantation genetic testing can be used to prevent reoccurrence. In addition, the use of prenatal genetic testing can allow patients with a family history of PIDDs to know if the fetus is affected. Prenatal knowledge of a genetically confirmed PIDD allows providers to prepare to provide support at birth for affected infants. When an affected patient has been diagnosed, it is important to determine the carrier status of their parents, if possible. In the case of novel mutations, the parents of the proband would not be at increased risk of having another child with that particular immunodeficiency. In addition, skewed lyonization of the X chromosome associated with manifestations of PIDDs has been described in female carriers of X-linked CGD,[12] hemophagocytic lymphohistiocytosis (HLH) due to mutations in *XIAP*,[13] and WAS.[14]

On a research level, the use of exploratory genetic testing in isolated, rare patients with severe manifestations of common infections or with rare infections has led to the discovery of novel molecular forms of immunodeficiency, the full clinical spectrum of which are yet to be defined.

LIMITATIONS OF GENETIC TESTING FOR PRIMARY IMMUNODEFICIENCY

Although genetic testing has immensely advanced immunology, not all patients can currently be genetically categorized. In fact, the use of next-generation sequencing panels has been associated with successful description of an underlying genetic diagnosis in 25% to 60% of those tested.[15,16] This is particularly true of patients carrying the diagnosis of common variable immunodeficiency (CVID). Genetic testing has helped to identify patients with complex syndromes of recurrent infections, autoimmunity, atopy, and autoinflammation, constituting immune dysregulatory disorders. Some families or individuals have monogenetic defects as the causative trigger for these symptoms; however, many patients remain without a genetic explanation for their symptoms.[17,18] It is possible, and perhaps even likely, that other factors, such as transcriptional signature differences or differences in DNA methylation (epigenetics),[19] may affect the disease manifestations. Regardless, treatment of patients with symptoms and laboratory findings suggestive of immunodeficiency should be treated symptomatically, rather than awaiting a definitive genetic diagnosis. A careful clinical history and physical examination to guide the choice of functional studies and genetic testing remains paramount to provide safe, effective, and personalized care in symptomatic patients.

OVERVIEW OF GENETIC TESTING MODALITIES
Chromosomal Microarray Analysis

Chromosomal microarray analysis (CMA), is also known as array comparative genomic hybridization. In this test, chromosomal losses and gains (copy number variants [CNVs]) throughout the genome are detected[20] by comparing the amount of DNA in a given region's hybridization intensities between the patient's DNA and a normal control.[21] Gene deletions and duplications of approximately 200 kb or 200,000 nucleotides can be identified by CMA. CMA allows the detection of CNVs, microdeletions, microduplications, and most unbalanced rearrangements of chromosome structure (translocations).[22,23] It may also detect excessive homozygosity, suggestive of consanguinity, with increased risk for recessive disease or imprinting disorders. CMA provides greater analytical sensitivity than karyotyping. However, CMA cannot detect small duplications or deletions within single-gene or point mutations. CMA is also useful when paired with WES or WGS data analysis[24] because it has the strength of detecting areas of excessive homozygosity and insertions and deletions, which may be missed by WES. Single nucleotide polymorphism (SNP) arrays, which are the gold standard for CMA, are very useful as an adjunct to a WES to ensure that CNVs are not contributing to a clinical phenotype; the 2 tests complement each other in their strengths and weaknesses. The 22q11 deletion syndrome, with a heterozygous loss of genetic material, is commonly diagnosed using CMA.

Single-Gene Sanger Sequencing

Single-gene Sanger sequencing, developed in the late 1970s, is a highly accurate form of genetic sequencing in which a primer binds to the genetic region of interest and, in the presence of the 4 nucleotides used in DNA construction, extends the primer using the existing DNA strand from the patient as a template. The creation of this complementary strand is stopped when fluorescent dye-labeled deoxynucleoside triphosphates are incorporated into the reaction of DNA strand elongation. This creates DNA fragments of varied length that can be used to read off the DNA sequence by linking together the last labeled base from the longest to the shortest strands. This leads to a base-by-base replication of the patient's DNA sequence, which is compared to a reference sequence.[25] Although it is expensive, laborious, and time consuming, it is a highly accurate form of genetic sequencing. It is able to detect point mutations in a coding sequence, as well as intronic mutations, and some deletions and duplications. However, some deletions may be missed and some intronic regions may also not be detected. In a PIDD with 1 implicated gene, single-gene Sanger sequencing is a reliable method for diagnosis; for example, sequencing of *BTK* in a male patient with a lack of immunoglobulins and B cells but otherwise normal T cells. Single-gene Sanger sequencing is also a reliable and cost-effective method for assessing family members of an affected patient with a known mutation. Finally, it is necessary for clinical confirmation of variants detected using WES.

Next-Generation Sequencing

Next-generation high-throughput DNA sequencing (NGS) refers to a group of sequencing platforms that, similar to Sanger sequencing, process fragments of DNA sequences derived from primers using patient DNA as a template; however, unlike Sanger sequencing, the process does not require use of gels for separation of the fragments. Instead, NGS uses a charge-coupled device camera to detect the fluorescent-labeled nucleotide bases on the replicating DNA strand.[26] Another advantage of NGS is the ability to perform genetic analysis on hundreds of samples at a time, which allows for higher expediency of result reporting. Base pair by base pair, NGS is less costly than Sanger sequencing; however, Sanger sequencing is more sensitive and less error prone.

Gene Panels

Gene panels, which test for variants in known monogenic forms of phenotypically similar PIDDs, such as SCID, CGD, and HLH, have been commercially developed for clinical use using both Sanger sequencing and NGS. The utility of gene panels is inherently limited due to the focus only on the list of included genes versus WES or WGS methods, which are unbiased techniques not restricted to a set list of target genes. In the last 10 years, with the advent of more NGS-based testing, an ever-expanding list of gene mutations associated with PIDDs has been identified. It is challenging for panels to be updated quickly enough to keep pace. In addition, with many gene panels, it may not easy to detect splice site or regulatory mutations in known genes due to the technical details of the procedure. Neither of these problems are an issue with WES. Currently, most gene panels are faster and cheaper than WES or WGS but this is expected to evolve over time as NGS WES or WGS strategies continue to become less expensive.

Whole Exome Sequencing

WES examines the approximately 1% of the human genome responsible for synthesized proteins that make up the human body (ie, the exons). Exomes are sequenced using oligonucleotide probes (baits) that bind to the exome and are then captured for sequencing. NGS techniques are used to sequence the set of fragments and the resulting short reads are assembled into the whole exome using complex computer algorithms. Ideally, WES is performed as a trio, including samples from the proband patient and both biologic parents, to allow determination of maternal or paternal inheritance. If a single (heterozygous) mutation is identified in a gene that is known to cause a similar phenotype in a homozygous state, deletion or duplication Sanger sequencing of the gene of interest is important to complete the evaluation because large deletions and duplications are not optimally detected in WES. If another exon in the second copy of the gene of interest is deleted, the patient would effectively be homozygous for the variant identified on WES. The paired use of an SNP array to detect larger deletions or duplications allows CNV evaluation and augments the clinical yield of WES testing.[24,27,28] The issue of accurate data interpretation has also been improved though new open-access bioinformatics tools, particularly to assist with CNV analysis from WES data.[29,30] However, Sanger sequencing as confirmatory testing and functional testing to validate a change in expected protein function (either loss or gain) is critically important before making treatment decisions based on the detection of novel variants.

As a nonbiased genetic testing approach, WES allows detection of nontraditional phenotypes with known genetic mutations or novel genetic mutations. In the first study of 250 consecutive WES, 21% of subjects had an underlying genetic defect identified, both in conditions with stable, classic phenotypes and those with variable, less predictable phenotypes.[31] In a recent report, in a large cohort of PIDD subjects, the diagnostic rate using WES approached 40%, with some further improvement in diagnostic yield when WES was paired with tandem CMA.[24] Currently, WES is used most commonly in assessment of patients with complex clinical phenotypes that may be seen in multiple known genetic forms of immunodeficiency.[19,32,33] In addition to the ability to detect both known and novel genetic mutations associated with the patient's immune phenotype, WES also assesses unrelated genetic pathways, such as genes associated with risks of neurologic disease, malignancy, or cardiovascular disease. Therefore, genetic counseling of patients and their families before and after WES is of critical importance.

Whole Genome Testing

Using similar technology as WES, WGS evaluates most of the 99% of nonexonic DNA content missed by WES. However, because the exon baits used to identify the exons for WES are based on prior knowledge, they are limited and can miss novel exons or poorly understood regions, and not completely cover the entire exome.[34] With WGS it is also possible to more confidently assess for noncoding variants (ie, intronic mutations, splice site mutations, and other regulatory nonexonic mutations), as well as deletions and duplications, that can be missed in WES testing. Theoretically, these additional data have the potential to yield novel diagnoses for families and patients with a PIDD. The limitations are the increased cost (though this is decreasing rapidly), analysis complexity, and time, as well as data storage needs. In addition, although knowledge of the genetics of human disease is continually expanding, understanding of the implications of variations in nonexonic DNA remain limited, so diagnosis may be delayed by scientific understanding of what constitutes a normal genomic sequence. With further technological and scientific progress, WGS seems likely to be the future of clinical genetic analysis of immunodeficiency.

TARGETED TREATMENTS BASED ON GENETICALLY DEFINED DISORDERS

As introduced previously, a major advantage to the use of genetic testing in PIDDs is the ability to personalize therapy for a patient based on their particular genetic form of disease.

The use of biologics in immunodeficiency is rapidly evolving. By determining the specific mechanism of disease, a rational approach to the application of these treatments in primary immunodeficiency is possible. Examples include successful clinical use of interleukin (IL)-1R blockade (anakinra) in the treatment of NLRP3–mediated autoinflammatory disorders, IL-6R blockade (tocilizumab) in the treatment of STAT3-GOF–mediated immune dysregulation, recombinant CTLA-4 (abatacept) in the treatment of CTLA-4 haploinsufficiency and LRBA deficiency,[35] JAK1-JAK2 signaling blockade (ruxolitinib) in the treatment of STAT1-GOF–mediated immune dysregulation,[36,37] inhibition of the p110δ catalytic subunit (leniolisib) in the treatment of PIK3CD-GOF–mediated immune dysfunction,[38] CXCR4 to CXCL12 binding blockade (plerixafor) in WHIM, and blockade of the p40 chain common to IL-12 and IL-23 (ustekinumab) in the treatment of leukocyte adhesion deficiency type 1.[36,38] In addition, other nonbiologic therapies can be used in a selected fashion, with greater expectations of successful clinical response, such as the use of rapamycin in the treatment of patients with PIK3CD-GOF mutations[38,39] and IPEX patients [40] and the use of high dose magnesium to improve NK cell function in patients with MAGT1 LOF mutations.[36]

In addition to therapies targeting the mechanism of action of the targeted gene, genetics can also help to prognosticate the outcome of long-standing therapy. For example, SCID has classically been treated with HSCT, regardless of phenotype (or genotype); however, there are clear differences in late effects of HSCT for SCID that are affected by genotype, including survival, durability of T-cell immune reconstitution, and B-cell function.[41–43] Patients with Artemis SCID are more likely to have growth failure and other late toxicities with exposure to alkylator-based conditioning regimens. In comparison, recombinase-activating gene (RAG) defects do not seem to increase susceptibility to DNA damage after exposure to alkylating agents (eg, Busulfan) and ionizing radiation.

Patients with SCID due to RAG1 or RAG2 defects and adenosine deaminase (ADA) defects have been shown to have poorer T-cell reconstitution after HSCT.[44] However, patients with defects in the common gamma chain of IL2R or JAK3 usually have engraftment of T cells with poor engraftment of B cells in the absence of pretransplant conditioning.[43] Patients with SCID due to mutations in CD3ʒ or IL7 receptor α chain are more likely to have functioning B cells despite a lack of donor chimerism, and are more likely to be able to discontinue immunoglobulin supplementation after transplant, even without conditioning.[41,43] SCID caused by mutations in *DCLREIC* (Artemis), *PRKDC*, *LIG4* (Ligase4), *NHEJI* (Cernunnos), and *NBS1* (Nijmegen breakage syndrome)[45] are associated with radiosensitivity and have an increase in early mortality associated with myeloablative conditioning before transplant. Enzyme replacement therapy is uniquely available as a bridge to definitive therapy for ADA-SCID. In addition to SCID, many other severe forms of combined immunodeficiency have been treated with HSCT. However, without knowledge of the underlying genetic defect, the ability to determine outcomes data is limited. There have recently been several reports describing the post-HSCT outcomes for other forms of genetically defined and clinically severe immunodeficiency, including reticular dysgenesis,[46] activated PI3Kδ syndrome,[47] hypomorphic IKBKG or NEMO mutations,[48] and LRBA deficiency,[49] to name just a few.

FUTURE CONSIDERATIONS

Although HSCT is currently the treatment of choice for severe immunodeficiencies that have a genetic defect in cells derived from hematopoietic precursors, this therapy is limited by donor availability, toxicity associated with preparative conditioning regimens, and the risk of developing graft-versus-host disease or graft rejection due to HLA-mismatches between the donor and recipient. To avoid these limitations, gene therapy and gene editing hold promise and are in development for several forms of PIDD.

In gene therapy, hematopoietic stem cells are harvested from the affected patient and the corrected gene is randomly introduced to the stem cells' DNA sequence using a viral vector. Thus, although the genetically defective sequence is not removed, a normal sequence is added to the stem cells' DNA. The corrected stem cells are then reinfused to the patient, typically after administration of preparative chemotherapy at doses lower than those used for standard HSCT. This allows for expression of the corrected gene product; however, this expression is not tightly regulated.[50] Although early trials of gene therapy were associated with insertional mutagenesis,[51–55] the latest generation of gene therapy vectors include self-inactivating lentiviral vectors and self-inactivating gammaretroviral vectors. These vectors have been used to treat patients with ADA-SCID, X-linked SCID, WAS, and X-linked CGD with clinical efficacy and without vector-related complications in nearly 10 years of follow-up. At the time of this writing, gene therapy is commercially available for ADA-SCID in Europe and has outcomes that compare very favorably to traditional treatment with HSCT.

In contrast, the process of gene editing uses specifically targeted endonucleases to repair genetic mutations, disrupt the function of a mutated gene, or insert a new gene specifically into a desired site of the mutant gene with homologous repair of the induced DNA break. This allows for use of the naturally occurring regulatory components of the target gene.[50] This is likely to be of benefit to correct genes associated with immunodeficiency in either a gain-of-function or loss-of-function state, and may be able to be used in vivo to correct defects in immunologically important cells or organs that are not derived from hematopoietic stem cells.

Although it is likely that genetic testing will continue to use the testing modalities described previously, it is likely that expanded use of WES and WGS will be readily available for clinical use. In addition, other forms of genetic testing, including assessment of epigenetic changes, RNA sequencing, and T-cell receptor (TCR) or B-cell receptor sequencing will emerge as clinical diagnostic tools.

Epigenetics, heritable genetic changes, such as DNA methylation patterns, transcription factor expression, histone and chromatic modification, and noncoding RNA, are not due to mutations in the DNA sequence but they can alter gene expression. Epigenetics have been postulated to have a role in modifying B-cell function, leading to differing manifestations of CVID.[56]

Messenger RNA sequencing (mRNA-Seq) has been used on a research basis to assess the transcriptome, including alternatively spliced transcripts, posttranscriptional modifications, gene fusion, SNPs, and/or changes in gene expression over time or following certain exposures or treatments. mRNA-Seq has been coupled with WES or WGS to attempt to better characterize a population with CVID.[57]

Some T-cell deficiencies causing autoimmunity are associated with oligoclonal T-cell populations, such as Omenn syndrome. The ability to test for this skewing is now clinically available, using spectratyping, which allows PCR amplification of variable regions in the CDR3 of the TCR; however, it is not highly precise. In the research setting, high-throughput sequencing of the TCR allows for higher resolution analysis of the CDR3.[58] By better understanding the normal, age-specific, distribution of TCRs it is possible that researchers and clinicians will be better able to understand T-cell antigen specificity and its role in autoimmunity and immunodeficiency.

SUMMARY

The rapid increase in clinical access to varied forms of genetic testing in the last 10 years has quickly expanded the recognition of the vast spectrum of molecular mechanisms behind the symptoms seen in patients affected by PIDD. This understanding has led to an enhanced ability to plan targeted therapeutic strategies that are more likely to be of clinical benefit for a given molecular mechanism than the empiric therapies used previously, which were typically trialed on a symptom-based rationale. In addition, when supplied with genetic data to support the mechanism of disease, clinical immunologists are better able to provide effective counseling to patients regarding their own prognosis and the risk of similar symptoms affecting their family members.

Both the American Academy of Allergy, Asthma, and Immunology and the Clinical Immunology Society support the use of genetic testing in the diagnosis and management of patients with primary immunodeficiency because it is expected that determining the molecular cause of the disease will often affect management.[59,60] Practicing clinical immunologists should have the necessary clinical knowledge to counsel patients regarding the use of genetic testing and to determine which genes should be considered, as well as the most reasonable testing modality to potentially determine a conclusive diagnosis.

In the future, it is likely that the options for genetic testing will expand. With this will come further improvements to better define the molecular causes of symptoms in PIDDs. With that knowledge, it is hoped that similar expansions in molecularly directed therapies will occur.

REFERENCES

1. Vetrie D, Vorechobsky I, Sideras P, et al. The gene involved in X-Linked Agammaglobulinemia is a member of the src family of protein-tyrosine kinases. Nature 1993;361:226–33.

2. Noguchi M, Yi H, Rosenblatt HM, et al. Interleukin-2 receptor gamma chain mutation results in X-linked severe combined immunodeficiency in humans. Cell 1993;73(1):147–57.
3. Derry JM, Ochs HD, Francke U. Isolation of a novel gene mutated in Wiskott-Aldrich syndrome. Cell 1994;78(4):635–44.
4. Picard C, Bobby Gaspar H, Al-Herz W, et al. International Union of Immunological Societies: 2017 primary immunodeficiency diseases committee report on inborn errors of immunity. J Clin Immunol 2018;38(1):96–128.
5. Myers LA, Patel DD, Puck JM, et al. Hematopoietic stem cell transplantation for severe combined immunodeficiency in the neonatal period leads to superior thymic output and improved survival. Blood 2002;99(3):872–8.
6. Kwan A, Abraham RS, Currier R, et al. Newborn screening for severe combined immunodeficiency in 11 screening programs in the United States. JAMA 2014; 312(7):729–38.
7. Kuhns D, Alvord WG, Heller T, et al. Residual NADPH oxidase and survival in chronic granulomatous disease. N Engl J Med 2010;363:2600–10.
8. Van den Berg JM, van Koppen E, Ahlin A, et al. Chronic granulomatous disease: the European Experience. PLoS One 2009;4:e5234.
9. Crowley B, Ruffner M, McDonald McGinn DM, et al. Variable immune deficiency related to deletion size in chromosome 22q11.2 deletion syndrome. Am J Med Genet A 2018. https://doi.org/10.1002/ajmg.a.38597.
10. Papa R, Doglio M, Lachmann HJ, et al, Paediatric Rheumatology International Trials Organisation (PRINTO) and the Eurofever Project. A web-based collection of genotype-phenotype associations in hereditary recurrent fevers from the Eurofever registry. Orphanet J Rare Dis 2017;12(1):167.
11. Tirosh I, Yamazaki T, Frugoni F, et al. Recombination activity of human RAG2 mutations and correlation with the clinical phenotype. J Allergy Clin Immunol 2018. https://doi.org/10.1016/j.jaci.2018.04.027.
12. Marciano BE, Zerbe CS, Falcone EL, et al. X-linked carriers of chronic granulomatous disease: illness, lyonization, and stability. J Allergy Clin Immunol 2018; 141(1):365–71.
13. Holle JR, Marsh RA, Holdcroft AM, et al. Hemophagocytic lymphohistiocytosis in a female patient due to a heterozygous XIAP mutation and skewed X chromosome inactivation. Pediatr Blood Cancer 2015;62(7):1288–90.
14. Parolini O, Ressmann G, Haas OA, et al. X-linked Wiskott-Aldrich syndrome in a girl. N Engl J Med 1998;338(5):291–5.
15. Biesecker LG, Green RC. Diagnostic clinical genome and exome sequencing. N Engl J Med 2014;370(25):2418–25.
16. Moens LN, Falk-Sörqvist E, Asplund AC, et al. Diagnostics of primary immunodeficiency diseases: a sequencing capture approach. PLoS One 2014;9(12): e114901.
17. Chinn IK, Eckstein OS, Peckham-Gregory EC, et al. Genetic and mechanistic diversity in pediatric hemophagocytic lymphohistiocytosis. Blood 2018. https://doi.org/10.1182/blood2017-11-814244.
18. Ma CA, Stinson JR, Zhang Y, et al. Germline hypomorphic CARD11 mutations in severe atopic disease. Nat Genet 2017;49(8):1192–201.
19. Kienzler AK, Hargreaves CE, Patel SY. The role of genomics in common variable immunodeficiency disorders. Clin Exp Immunol 2017;188(3):326–32.
20. Zarrei M, MacDonald JR, Merico D, et al. A copy number variation map of the human genome. Nat Rev Genet 2015;16:172–83.

21. Bi W, Borgan C, Pursley AN, et al. Comparison of chromosome analysis and chromosomal microarray analysis: what is the value of chromosome analysis in today's genomic array era? Genet Med 2013;15:450–7.

22. Kang S, Shaw C, Ou Z, et al. Insertional translocation detected using FISH confirmation of array-comparative genomic hybridization (aCGH) results. Am J Med Genet A 2010;152A:1111–26.

23. Neill NJ, Ballif BC, Lamb AN, et al. Recurrence, submicroscopic complexity, and potential clinical relevance of copy gains detected by array CGH that are shown to be unbalanced insertions by FISH. Genome Res 2011;21(4):535–44.

24. Stray-Pedersen A, Sorte HS, Samarakoon P, et al. Primary immunodeficiency diseases: genomic approaches delineate heterogeneous Mendelian disorders. J Allergy Clin Immunol 2017;139:232–45.

25. Sanger F, Nicklen S, Coulsen AR. DNA sequencing with chain terminating inhibitors. Proc Natl Acad Sci U S A 1977;74(2):5463–7.

26. Ansorge WJ. Next-generation DNA sequencing techniques. N Biotechnol 2009; 25(4):195–203.

27. Cirulli ET, Goldstein DB. Uncovering the roles of rare variants in common disease through whole-genome sequencing. Nat Rev Genet 2010;11(6):415–25.

28. Retterer K, Scuffins J, Schmidt D, et al. Assessing copy number from exome sequencing and exome array CGH based on CNV spectrum in a large clinical cohort. Genet Med 2015;17:623–9.

29. Magi A, Tattini L, Cifola I, et al. EXCAVATOR: detecting copy number variants from whole- Keller exome sequencing data. Genome Biol 2013;14:R120.

30. Fromer M, Purcell SM. Using XHMM software to detect copy number variation in whole-exome sequencing data. Curr Protoc Hum Genet 2014;81:7.23.1-21.

31. Yang Y, Muzny DM, Reid JG, et al. Clinical whole-exome sequencing for the diagnosis of mendelian disorders. N Engl J Med 2013;369(16):1502–11.

32. Amininejad L, Charloteaux B, Theatre E, et al, International IBD Genetics Consortium. Analysis of genes associated with monogenic primary immunodeficiency identifies rare variants in XIAP in patients with Crohn's disease. Gastroenterology 2018;154(8):2165–77.

33. Mukda E, Trachoo O, Pasomsub E, et al. Exome sequencing for simultaneous mutation screening in children with hemophagocytic lymphohistiocytosis. Int J Hematol 2017;106(2):282–90.

34. Chou J, Ohsumi TK, Geha RS. Use of whole exome and genome sequencing in the identification of genetic causes of primary immunodeficiencies. Curr Opin Allergy Clin Immunol 2012;12:623–6.

35. Lo B, Zhang K, Lu W, et al. Patients with LRBA deficiency show CTLA4 loss and immune dysregulation responsive to abatacept therapy. Science 2015; 349(6246):436–40.

36. Marciano BE, Holland SM. Primary immunodeficiency diseases: current and emerging therapeutics. Front Immunol 2017;8:937.

37. Weinacht KG, Charbonnier LM, Alroqi F, et al. Ruxolitinib reverses dysregulated T helper cell responses and controls autoimmunity caused by a novel signal transducer and activator of transcription 1 (STAT1) gain-of-function mutation. J Allergy Clin Immunol 2017;139(5):1629–40.e2.

38. Notarangelo LD, Fleisher TA. Targeted strategies directed at the molecular defect: toward precision medicine for select primary immunodeficiency disorders. J Allergy Clin Immunol 2017;139(3):715–23.

39. Lucas CL, Kuehn HS, Zhao F, et al. Dominant-activating germline mutations in the gene encoding the PI(3)K catalytic subunit p110δ result in T cell senescence and human immunodeficiency. Nat Immunol 2014;15(1):88–97.

40. Yong PL, Russo P, Sullivan KE. Use of sirolimus in IPEX and IPEX-like children. J Clin Immunol 2008;28(5):581–7.

41. Haddad E, Leroy S, Buckley RH. B-cell reconstitution for SCID: should a conditioning regimen be used in SCID treatment? J Allergy Clin Immunol 2013;131: 994–1000.

42. Heimall J, Puck J, Buckley R, et al. Current knowledge and priorities for future research in late effects after hematopoietic stem cell transplantation (HCT) for severe combined immunodeficiency patients: a consensus statement from the second pediatric blood and marrow transplant consortium international conference on late effects after pediatric HCT. Biol Blood Marrow Transplant 2017;23(3): 379–87.

43. Buckley RH, Win CM, Moser BK, et al. Post-transplantation B cell function in different molecular types of SCID. J Clin Immunol 2013;33:96–110.

44. Sarzotti-Kelsoe M, Win CM, Parrott RE, et al. Thymic output, T cell diversity and T-cell function in long term human SCID chimeras. Blood 2009;114:1445–53.

45. Cowan MJ, Gennery AC. Radiation-sensitive severe combined immunodeficiency: the arguments for and against conditioning before hematopoietic cell transplantation – what to do? J Allergy Clin Immunol 2015;136:1178–85.

46. Hoenig M, Lagresle-Peyrou C, Pannicke U, et al, European Society for Blood and Marrow Transplantation (EBMT) Inborn Errors Working Party. Reticular dysgenesis: international survey on clinical presentation, transplantation, and outcome. Blood 2017;129(21):2928–38.

47. Okano T, Imai K, Tsujita Y, et al. Hematopoietic stem cell transplantation for progressive combined immunodeficiency and lymphoproliferation in activated PI3Kd syndrome type 1. J Allergy Clin Immunol 2018. [Epub ahead of print].

48. Miot C, Imai K, Imai C, et al. Hematopoietic stem cell transplantation in 29 patients hemizygous for hypomorphic IKBKG/NEMO mutations. Blood 2017; 130(12):1456–67.

49. Seidel MG, Böhm K, Dogu F, et al, Inborn Errors Working Party of the European Group for Blood and Marrow Transplantation. Treatment of severe forms of LPS-responsive beige-like anchor protein deficiency with allogeneic hematopoietic stem cell transplantation. J Allergy Clin Immunol 2018;141(2):770–5.

50. Kohn DB, Kuo CY. New frontiers in the therapy of primary immunodeficiency: from gene addition to gene editing. J Allergy Clin Immunol 2017;139(3):726–32.

51. Hacein-Bey-Abina S, von Kalle C, Schmidt M, et al. A serious adverse event after successful gene therapy for X-linked severe combined immunodeficiency. N Engl J Med 2003;348:255–6.

52. Hacein-Bey-Abina S. LMO2-associated clonal T cell proliferation in two patients after gene therapy for SCID-X1. Science 2003;302:415–9.

53. Fischer A, Abina SH, Thrasher A, et al. LMO2 and gene therapy for severe combined immunodeficiency. N Engl J Med 2004;350:2526–7.

54. Howe SJ, Mansour MR, Schwarzwaelder K, et al. Insertional mutagenesis combined with acquired somatic mutations causes leukemogenesis following gene therapy of SCID-X1 patients. J Clin Invest 2008;118:3143–50.

55. Stein S, Ott MG, Schultze-Strasser S, et al. Genomic instability and myelodysplasia with monosomy 7 consequent to EVI1activation after gene therapy for chronic granulomatous disease. Nat Med 2010;16:198–204.

56. Rae W. Indications to epigenetic dysfunction in the pathogenesis of common variable immunodeficiency. Arch Immunol Ther Exp (Warsz) 2017;65(2):101–10.

57. van Schouwenburg PA, Davenport EE, Kienzler AK, et al. Application of whole genome and RNA sequencing to investigate the genomic landscape of common variable immunodeficiency disorders. Clin Immunol 2015;160(2):301–14.

58. Wong GK, Heather JM, Barmettler S, et al. Immune dysregulation in immunodeficiency disorders: the role of T-cell receptor sequencing. J Autoimmun 2017;80: 1–9.

59. Bonilla FA, Khan DA, Ballas ZK, et al. Practice parameter for the diagnosis and management of primary immunodeficiency. J Allergy Clin Immunol 2015;136: 1186–205.

60. Heimall JR, Hagin D, Hajjar J, et al. Use of genetic testing for primary immunodeficiency patients. J Clin Immunol 2018;38(3):320–9.

Printed and bound by CPI Group (UK) Ltd, Croydon, CR0 4YY

03/10/2024

01040391-0012